C0-ASC-329

Acupressure
Yoga &
YOU

ACUPRESSURE YOGA and YOU

By Louise Taylor & Betty Bryant

Japan Publications, Inc.

Copyright © 1984 by Louise Taylor and Betty Bryant
All rights reserved, including the right to reproduce this book or portions
thereof in any form without the written permission of the publisher.

*This health care system is not meant to replace medical diagnosis or treatment.
If symptoms are severe or persistent, you should always consult your physician.*

Published by JAPAN PUBLICATIONS, INC., Tokyo and New York

Distributors:
UNITED STATES: *Kodansha International/USA, Ltd., through Harper & Row,
Publishers, Inc., 10 East 53rd Street, New York, New York 10022.* SOUTH
AMERICA: *Harper & Row, Publishers, Inc., International Department.* CANADA:
Fitzhenry & Whiteside Ltd., 150 Lesmil Road, Don Mills, Ontario M3B 2T6.
MEXICO AND CENTRAL AMERICA: *HARLA S. A. de C. V., Apartado 30–546,
Mexico 4, D. F.* BRITISH ISLES: *International Book Distributors Ltd., 66 Wood
Lane End, Hemel Hempstead, Herts HP2 4RG.* EUROPEAN CONTINENT:
*Fleetbooks, S. A., c/o Feffer and Simons (Nederland) B. V., Rijnkade 170,
1382 GT Weesp, The Netherlands.* AUSTRALIA AND NEW ZEALAND: *Book
Wise, 1 Jeanes Street, Beverley, South Australia 5009*
THE FAR EAST AND JAPAN: *Japan Publications Trading Co., Ltd., 1–2–1,
Sarugaku-cho, Chiyoda-ku, Tokyo 101.*

First edition: May 1984

LCCC No. 84–080639
ISBN 0–87040–574–8

Printed in U.S.A.

Preface

The aim of this book is to stimulate the reader's interest in an alternative approach to personal health care. Acupressure and yoga provide a valuable resource for anyone making the transition to a more self-directed health style. Acupressure is based on the understanding that organic disorders are reflected at certain points on the body. Sustained pressure at these points relieves pathological symptoms and balances and rejuvenates the whole system. Yoga asanas, by their very nature, also balance and rejuvenate the body. Together, acupressure and yoga stimulate the body's natural powers of revitalization, eliminate fatigue and promote a sense of health and well-being. It has been found that by combining the two disciplines the effectiveness of both is enhanced and accelerated.

This book presents an alternative way to deal with many discomforts. Rather than reaching for relief through medication, you may, instead, take a self-initiated step toward promoting symptomatic relief of health problems. There are no side effects concomitant with this form of health care, such as muscular pain (often experienced after strenuous activity), undue fatigue or allergic reactions. There are no age limits. Younger people will find through this dynamic combination a means by which to maintain and increase bodily strength and flexibility. Older people will find that acupressure and yoga can prevent many of the problems associated with aging.

As you become more open to taking charge of your health and well-being, you will open the door to a new and rewarding experience. A minimum amount of practice will allow you to easily take more initiative in bringing personal health care within your own sphere of influence. The book is arranged so that you can go through it systematically or you can use any one section as it particularly applies to your needs or interests. If you are consistent in your practice you will find that this program becomes easy and fun to do.

Acupressure and yoga are both ancient healing arts. Both are thousands of years old and have proven to be effective for the millions of people who practice them. They are both safe treatments, readily available, inexpensive and based on principles of order, balance and self-reliance. They are offered in this book as an antidote for the mental and physical tension caused by the fast pace of Western living.

The Eastern healing arts are based on two basic beliefs. One is the belief in the inevitablity of change. The other is in the self renewing and self healing capacity of nature. Eastern thought holds that man and nature are one and the same. Fluctuations in health are experienced by everyone and can be expected as part of the natural order. Seasons change with regularity, and just as nature is self renewing, people need only to learn that they also have the natural capacity to renew and revitalize their bodies. In using the healing arts of yoga and acupressure, you will learn to release your own healing potential and achieve a high level of wellness.

This book was written because we would like everyone to be able to share what we have found to be a valuable and rewarding experience. Both of us have taught acupressure and yoga classes for a number of years. As an experiment, we taught one class combining the two disciplines. We found that our students thoroughly enjoyed the combination. They were able to easily assimilate the knowledge and skill from both traditions. Their sense of self-awareness and personal growth was wonderful to see. Many achieved a higher level of wellness and were able to overcome what they previously had thought to be chronic disabilities. The techniques presented in this book are for anyone who feels the need to take an active part in, and claim responsibility for, his or her personal health and well-being.

Acknowledgment

Our sincere and grateful thanks to Art Taylor and Bill Bryant for their patience and constructive criticism throughout the preparation of this book. To Colleen Davis-Niemi who posed for the pictures and shared her expertise as a Yoga teacher.

Our thanks also go to Stef Butler who helped with the photographs and to Norma Bouweraerts who took time out from her busy schedule to prepare the diagrams. To Donna Taylor for excellent advice, to Janet Denison for hours of proofreading, and to Sandra Taylor for her popcorn.

Contents

1. *Acupressure, Yoga and You*

Acupressure and Yoga: A Perfect Blend

Acupressure and yoga complement each other in many ways. When you are practicing yoga, you are naturally stimulating, sedating or balancing the acupressure meridians. When you understand the nature of the meridians you will be able to utilize acupressure and yoga together to formulate a wellness program based upon your individual needs.

When you begin your practice you will find that most of your concentration is spent on learning to correctly execute the yoga asanas and locating the acupressure points. This is a necessary first step associated with any kind of learning process. After you become thoroughly familiar with the postures and can easily find the acupressure points to use, your practice will become smoother and less self-conscious. In this stage you will become more self-aware and more able to let yourself feel the benefits of each stretch and the action of each acupressure point. As you progressively master the asanas and can locate the pressure points with ease, you will no longer have to concentrate on what you are doing and you will be able to experience a state of mind-body consciousness that is similar to meditation where the total experience transcends the separate parts of each movement. When you practice yoga and acupressure, you will become extremely aware of your body and your feelings. You will learn to trust your own judgment and vary your pace in a flexible combination of stretches and pressure point techniques. You will deeply, but gently, release your tensions, let yourself relax completely and become more aware of a developing harmony and unity throughout your body.

Some of the many ways you will find the combination of acupressure and yoga to be beneficial are:

Stress Reduction: Stress and tension block the flow of energy in the body's meridian system. Both yoga and acupressure release these blocks of energy.

Balance: For the balance of the physical, mental, emotional and spiritual bodies, energy must flow smoothly through all of the meridians. Yoga, combined with a conscious use of acupressure points, allows this energy to flow smoothly.

Greater Body Awareness and Understanding: Working with acupressure and yoga brings greater understanding and awareness in all areas of body function.

Relaxation: Both of these systems promote deep relaxation. Through the practice of acupressure each part of the body can be sedated as needed. Relaxation is an integral part of yoga, combining deep relaxation and breathing exercises.

Vibrant Health Each Day: The goal of both of these systems is to promote good health and allow you to live each day fully.

Introduction to Acupressure

Thousands of years before American and European scientists discovered atoms, electrons and electricity, the Chinese developed a concept of the entire universe as being in balance between negative (Yin) and positive (Yang) energy forces. Yin and Yang represent the negative and positive dualism existing within all things, from the protons and electrons of the atoms to the seasonal changes and all of the opposite or opposing forces in nature. This duality is fundamental in both ancient Chinese and modern scientific thought. An understanding of this concept is helpful in working with acupressure.

It is not necessary to accept Chinese philosophical concepts in order to learn acupressure (the actual meaning of acupressure is finger pressure). We can, however, use the formulas they have worked out over the centuries for relieving pain and disabilities in various parts of the body. The human body was seen by the ancient Chinese to be a microcosm of the universe requiring a balance of Yin and Yang energy to function properly. Over 3,000 years ago these principles were written down in the *I Ching* or *The Book of Change.*

The Chinese also developed the concept of "vital energy" which is called "Chi." This energy is even finer than electrical energy. It is the fundamental energy of the universe and it enters the human body through the breath and through the intake of food. Food and air then combine to form the life energy of every living being.

Vital energy is seen by practitioners of Oriental medicine to have a definite predictable route throughout the body. It flows along pathways that traverse the body in a fixed pattern somewhat like the network of a complex railway system. The energy travels along this network in pathways divided into major routes called meridians. These meridians were named for the organ or function served by each section of the pathway. On these routes there are numerous "tiny points" where the energy comes to the surface of the body. These points are called acupuncture or acupressure points.

This system was first made public 4,000 years ago in what may be the first medical book ever written, *The Yellow Emperor's Classic of Internal Medicine* or simply the *Yellow Emperor's Classic.* It is interesting to note that modern electronic instruments now enable us to locate acupuncture/acupressure points precisely where the ancient Chinese showed them to be. These points respond to any change in the flow of vital energy. They appear to act somewhat like resistors in an electrical current by adjusting the speed and power of the flow. The response is a kind of fluid elasticity which tightens or slackens as necessary. It is through the meridians and acupressure points that the vital energy reaches the organs. If the organ or gland, nourished by a particular flow, is not functioning properly, points along the meridian will be painful or stiff. By reestablishing the energy flow along this organ's pathway, the organ or gland will be revitalized and health restored. The meridians can also be thrown off balance by the tensions and stresses of modern life. When this happens, the flow of vital energy becomes blocked, too intense, or too weak resulting in the development of disorders in the function of the body.

In this book, we have focused on the particular points along the meridians which are used to bring the body into balance by stimulating, sedating, or balancing the energy. There are many points along each meridian but you will derive great benefit from learning just three points on each one. These points are easily found and they lend themselves well to fingertip stimulation because of their pressure responsive nature.

The purpose of stimulating a meridian is to bring a fresh supply of energy to that particular meridian which is low or deficient in energy. When energy is lacking in a meridian, the organ involved as well as the muscles and nerves are working at a deficient level. This can ultimately have an adverse effect upon the vitality of the entire body. Stimulating the specific point, designated in each chapter, will generate a revitalization of that particular energy flow and thereby remove blocks or dams in the organ's system which could have prevented a state of good health.

In each chapter you will find a list of symptoms which are related to a loss of energy within a specific meridian. By holding the stimulation point whenever possible during your asana practice or while in a seated position, after you have completed the stretches, the effect of the stimulation point will be enhanced. To aid in the process of stimulation, press the point firmly and hold it for about two minutes.

Sedation is the process of quieting or draining off excess energy which has been trapped or blocked within a particular meridian. These blocks occur when stress and tension contract the muscles and tighten the nerves. Pressure on the sedation point of each meridian has the effect of re-distributing blocked energy. When energy is blocked it causes a depletion in another part of the body. Too much energy in a particular meridian can also cause the corresponding organ to malfunction, sometimes causing pain along the meridian's route.

In each chapter you will find a list of symptoms which are related to an overabundance of energy within a specific meridian. By holding a sedation point whenever possible during your asana practice, or while in a seated position after you have completed the stretches, the effect of the sedation point will be enhanced. To aid in the process of sedation, press the point lightly and hold it for about two minutes.

The function of the balancing point within each meridian is to evenly dis-tribute that meridian's energy. It also provides energy to the organ specifically related to the meridian. Therefore, this point automatically reestablishes the meridian's energy balance whether the meridian energy is excessive (blocked) or deficient (lacking or low).

The balancing point for each meridian is given in the designated chapter. It is a good point to use for balancing and maintaining a healthy flow of energy in the body. To promote good health, press each specific balancing point whenever possible during your asana practice or while in a seated position after you have completed the stretches. The pressure point should be held with moderate pressure for one to two minutes while maintaining a relaxed state of mind.

Besides stimulating, sedating and balancing the meridian, great benefit is also derived by massaging the entire meridian lightly with finger pressure, stopping to work longer where there is pressure or distress. We instinctively know which places on our body to rub when we are experiencing discomfort. The body has its own system for safeguarding its health. If your eyes feel tired, you rub them. We wring our hands when we feel anxious and if we have a headache, we frequently rub our temples or the sides of the head. In so doing we contact many of the pressure points that bring relief. Whenever we are hurt, we involuntarily massage the pain away just as when a child falls, he instinctively rubs the area that causes pain.

There are several forms of acupressure that are being practiced today. They all use finger pressure to balance, stimulate and release energy from the specific points along the meridian pathways but the method of approach is different for each one. The main types of acupressure include:

Shiatsu: Shiatsu uses a series of points which are pressed for a few seconds in a vigorous fashion. The points run consecutively along a flow of energy and the pressure should be firm. It is usually done by a therapist.

Do-In: Do-In acupressure is self-acupressure. It includes a set of stretching exercises as well as self-massage at specific points. It also includes a set of breathing exercises and incorporates these with the exercises to form a daily program of practice.

G-Jo: G-Jo, or acupressure for first aid, utilizes specific points in response to symptomatic needs. In this type of acupressure it is necessary to be aware of the specific points that act to relieve the discomfort, injury or disease of each part of the body.

Jin Shin: Jin Shin acupressure uses prolonged finger pressure. It focuses on the balancing of the meridians and correct function of the organs. It uses the pressure of two points at one time which stimulates the flow of energy between two points. It can be self-administered or done by a therapist.

All of these forms of acupressure can be perfectly blended with other disciplines such as yoga because they focus on the balance of the body and awakening of the spirit.

Introduction to Yoga

Yoga originated in ancient India. It is over 6,000 years old. Begun by Tibetan monks, the techniques and theories were initially handed down orally by a chain of teachers and students. Later on they were written down. The first written account is attributed to the Indian sage Patanjali, who codified the complete system of Yoga in the 2nd century B.C. The *Yoga Sutras* remains as one of India's most important writings. Patanjali chose 84 main postures from the thousands then in use. In India today these same postures are basic to the study of Yoga.

The word *Yoga* is derived from the Sanskrit root verb "yuj," which means to join or unite. It signifies the joining of the individual with the universal reality. It also means the union of the conscious mind with the deeper levels of the unconscious which results in a totally integrated personality. Just as Acupressure seeks perfect balance in the human body, the yogic ideal of unification is called "mukusha" and connotes a perfect balance or state or naturalness. It cannot be too strongly stressed that the whole of life strives towards this ideal, which is described by the Christian religion as "the peace which passeth all understanding." When we begin to search for balance and natural harmony in our own lives, we begin to grow on a path that leads to deeper understanding and fulfillment. At such a time we learn that satisfaction comes from something which we find to be deep within and does not rely on external stimulation. In the sixth Chapter of the *Bhagavad Gita*, which is the most important authority on Yoga philosophy, Krishna explains to Arjuna the meaning of Yoga as a deliverance from the sorrows of this world.

"When his mind, intellect and self are under control, freed from restless desire, so that they rest in the spirit within, a man becomes a Yukta—one in communion with God. A lamp does not flicker in a place where no winds blow; so it is with a Yogi, who controls his mind, intellect and self, being absorbed in the spirit within him. When the restlessness of the mind, intellect and self is stilled through the practice of Yoga, the Yogi, by the grace of the spirit within himself, finds fulfillment. Then he knows the joy eternal which is beyond the pale of the senses which his reason cannot grasp. He abides in this reality and moves not therefrom. He has found the treasure above all others. There is nothing higher than this. He who has achieved it, shall not be moved by the greatest sorrow."

This is the real meaning of Yoga—a deliverance from contact with pain and sorrow.

Although basic to all existence, balance is often upset. Yoga attempts to restore it through a threefold path of development; physical, mental and spiritual. Yoga claims that there is no artificial separation between that which is body and that which is mind. This is the logic behind the fact that all its teachings begin with the physical, with *Hatha Yoga*, the philosophy of physical well-being. The goals of acupressure and the goals of Hatha Yoga are the same, to gain control of the body's energy flow and to direct it in positive, healing ways. The vital energy called "Chi" by the Chinese and "Ki" by the Japanese is called "prana" in India. *Prana* is seen to be everywhere and in everything; it is the basic force that animates all matter. In the study of Yoga the life force or prana is closely associated with breathing practices which control and direct this important energy. Freed and able to flow throughout the body, it can stimulate both body and mind; blocked and distorted, it can sap and deplete our activities.

The postures and breathing techniques of Hatha Yoga combine to provide vitality and well-being. Each of the postures is enhanced by the addition of proper breathing (*Pranayama*). The stretches, breathing techniques, and deep relaxation exercises of Hatha Yoga balance and tone the entire body. They provide an effective method for dealing with our normal fast paced lives and give quick and observable results in relieving stress and tension.

The name Hatha is made up of two Sanskrit roots "Ha," which stands for the sun, and "tha" for the moon. In the science of Hatha Yoga the right side of the body is the positive, male, sun, heat side. The left side of the body is the negative, female, moon, cool side. This corresponds to the Oriental theory of yin and yang. Through the practice of Hatha Yoga the two sides of the body and their characteristic forces are brought into balance. By practicing Hatha Yoga, one can obtain physical health, mental clarity and steady strength of mind and character. The practice and eventual mastery of the Hatha Yoga postures and breathing patterns results in a balanced and steady mind and body. Hatha Yoga asanas (in the Sanskrit language *asana* means bench or steady position) are designed to give maximum flexibility and strength to the skeletal, muscular and nervous systems. Asanas stretch and strengthen the spine and work, with the aid of breathing exercises, to balance and revitalize the body. While doing the stretches of Hatha Yoga the vital organs are massaged and blood circulation is increased. The asanas are practiced not only to achieve a state of well-being but as a preparation for meditation. To meditate effectively, it is important to have a strong, flexible body that is able to remain in a meditative posture for long periods without becoming fatigued.

You will notice that the Yoga asanas are named for animals and natural phenomenon. The reason for this can be found in the *Vedas*, ancient Hindu scriptures, which describe how Yoga exercises were created and designed by the king of Yogis, Lord *Shiva*, at the beginning of time. Lord Shiva observed how the animal kingdom remained strong and healthy in harsh and varied environments. After studying their breathing and sleeping patterns as well as their movements, he isolated the underlying techniques which enabled them to survive efficiently and, using these techniques, developed the Hatha Yoga system.

Aside from Hatha Yoga, there are several interconnected branches or paths which the student of Yoga can choose to follow. Each of these paths lead to personal development and eventually to a state of higher consciousness where the individual self merges with the Universal Self bringing man and nature into complete harmony. Many serious students of yoga choose more than one path. Swami Vivekananda, who was instrumental in introducing Yoga to the United States around the turn of the century, believed in a synthesis of the various Yogas to achieve self-discovery. Others believe that it is more beneficial to follow one path to their goal.

The other paths of Yoga are:

Mantra Yoga: A *mantra* is a repeated phrase. *Japa* is the term used to describe the actual repetition. Therefore, Mantra Yoga is sometimes called *Japa Yoga.* Followers of Mantra Yoga repeat certain mantras thousands of times. A mantra takes the place of usual thought patterns and focuses the mind on the vibration of the mantra. The mantra and the goal of the mantra merge and become one and the same.

Bhakti Yoga: Bhakti Yoga involves concentration and meditation on the Divine. It is the Yoga of faith, devotion and worship. A lover of art, music, or nature is practicing Bhakti Yoga whether or not he calls it by that name. Service toward man and animals and an unselfish striving to see the Universal Principle in all things is the path of one practicing this Yoga. Bhakti Yoga is often combined with Mantra Yoga. Chanting the mantra with love, the Yogi becomes inspired and filled with bliss.

Karma Yoga: This is the Yoga of action. Its name comes from the Sanskrit "kri" which means "to do." It is based on the law of cause and effect, with good deeds producing good results. The follower of *Karma Yoga* feels that he is a necessary unit in the whole process of life.

Jnana Yoga: In Sanskrit "jnana" means "to know." This is the path of knowledge or intellectual attainment. The truths of existence and the nature of the Self are examined. In this Yoga the student focuses on himself not as the body, feelings, personality, or intellect, but as their user. This Yoga raises the seeker above limitations and attempts to recognize the similarities and truths in all philosophies.

Raja Yoga: *Raja* signifies "royal or kingly." This is the Yoga of self-mastery through mental control. It seeks to gain control over the stream of thoughts that flow through the mind. It attempts to check that flow and still the mind by means of concentration (*Dharana*) and contemplation (*Dhyana*). By these practices a state of Superconsciousness (*Samadhi*) may be reached. *Raja Yoga* is closely linked with Hatha Yoga. The two are often practiced together. Hatha Yoga aims at mastering the body and Raja Yoga aims at mastering the mind.

Laya Yoga: This term, meaning "latency" in the sense of "hidden," defines a type of Yoga applied to the stilling of the mind in order to awaken and direct the inner force called *Kundalini.* The kundalini is seen as a "life-force" which purifies the body by traveling through each of the body's energy centers (*chakras*).

Getting Started

This book has been designed to present the complex disciplines of acupressure and Yoga in a simple and understandable way. Before you start to work with the material presented you should take a few moments to design a program that will fit your specific needs. To derive the most benefit from your daily practice you will need to properly prepare your physical surroundings and set a mental climate that will be most conducive to your success. If you begin your study of *Acupressure, Yoga and You* with a few basic concepts clearly in mind, you will be better prepared to achieve your goals.

Mental Guidelines

Intuition: Everyone has an "inner knowing" or a sense self which we call intuition. Most of us, in our modern culture, are not attuned to this creative principle although it is operating at all times in our life. Our tendency is to become more aware of external stimuli and less aware of the internal processes that occur. Part of the discipline of Acupressure and Yoga is to quiet the mind and allow one's self to become aware of this inner resource. As you practice the postures in combination with the pressure points of the body, various thoughts and feelings will arise. As you learn to focus on these thoughts and feelings you will gain new insights and understandings about your total being.

Self-Discipline: Our modern world provides a variety of distractions and interests which can seem more urgent than a course of self-study. Our natural resistance to discipline is ingrained in our society with its emphasis on play and recreation. All of us need to take time, however, for contemplation and growth. Discipline is necessary in any worthwhile endeavor and is the only way to produce lasting and valuable rewards. A lasting reward is to be found by spending just a few minutes a day with Acupressure and Yoga. At first it may seem difficult, however, after a few weeks of continued practice you will find that many improvements have occurred in your health and well-being. As you learn to work with the meridians to alleviate symptomatic conditions and have become more flexible and graceful through practicing the asanas, you will begin to find greater motivation to continue the discipline of your daily practice.

Concentration: In order to derive maximum benefit from your program, you should set the stage mentally as well as physically. Your mental outlook can make the difference in the effectiveness of your practice. You will find, at first, that you may experience difficulty in remaining mentally centered or focused for any length of time. This is usual when beginning a study of

Acupressure or Yoga. By gently reminding yourself to fully concentrate on the location of a pressure point, a breathing technique, or the stretch of an asana, you will gradually find that your mind remains focused for longer and longer periods of time. The extraneous thoughts that pass through your mind should be allowed to come and go. Thoughts will only linger if you allow them to. The thoughts that you choose to think during your practice can determine the success of your activity.

Positive Thinking: You should not only attempt to center your mind when you practice, but you should also hold a positive attitude about the results that you wish to achieve. A positive attitude will enhance your new skills and can carry over from your practice into many areas of your daily life. Promoting a sense of self-worth is an important adjunct to the success of any new endeavor. It is also extremely vital for establishing new patterns leading to optimum health.

Physical Guidelines

Time: Set aside a half hour each day for your practice. As you become more proficient in remembering the asanas you will need a shorter time for the same number of stretches. It is always best to determine in advance how much time you have to complete your program. If possible, exercise at the same time each day. In the morning you will not be as limber as you are in the afternoon or evening. The morning stretches will help you to feel better all day, while in the evening the stretches will relax you in preparation for a good sleep.

Place: Exercise in the same place each time. You should make sure that you have good ventilation and that the room temperature is comfortable. Telephones, radio, television or other distractions should be put aside during your practice. You will need adequate space to exercise comfortably and a rug to lie on or a blanket folded in four to protect you from the hardness of the floor. A spongy or air filled mattress may cause an injury.

Clothing: Wear clean, light clothing that is loose and comfortable. If you prefer, tights and a leotard will make you more aware of the movements of your body. Remove your wristwatch, glasses and any jewelry you may be wearing.

General Health: You should wait at least an hour after eating to begin your exercises.

Consult your doctor about the exercises if you have any of the following: high blood pressure, dizziness, detached retina, ulcers, hernia, fractured bones, or are more than three months pregnant. Women who are menstruating should not do the inverted postures.

2. How to Use the Book

Working with the Book

By using this book you will gradually begin to experience greater health naturally. Not only is it important to design your own health care system, it is rewarding to experience an increase in energy and relief from symptoms without the use of aspirin or other chemicals. With greater self-reliance you will be more confident of continuing good health for a lifetime. Keep in mind the Oriental point of view that healing depends upon attunement with the cyclic ebb and flow of one's own vital energy.

Combining Acupressure and Yoga: In combining Acupressure and Yoga you will be working with two powerful and time tested health enhancement methods. Both are thousands of years old and are based in the belief that man, as a part of nature, has the capacity for self regeneration and self renewal. By releasing energy blockages, these two systems combine synergistically to bring about new and renewed vitality. The following information is presented to enable you to work effectively in blending Acupressure and Yoga into a total health care system.

It is important to start your program with a complete warm-up. The sequence of exercises in Chapter 3 will provide the stretching and flexibility necessary to achieve maximum benefits and to prevent injury.

In each Chapter, 4 through 17, you will find:

1. An explanation of the meridian, what it is and what it does.
2. A diagram of the meridian's flow on the body with an arrow indicating the direction of the energy flow.
3. Points along the meridian you will be using.
4. Some common symptoms that are related to the malfunction of the meridian.
5. Procedure for stimulating, sedating or balancing each meridian.
6. Six asanas to use in combination with each meridian.

When designing your program, first look through Chapters 4 through 17 of the book to identify your individual needs. Become familiar with the advantages of using several of the asanas within a particular practice period to balance your body in general or to relieve several symptoms of discomfort. You can combine asanas from more than one of the fourteen chapters into a single program to best fit your total body needs.

Write Out Your Program: When you have clearly defined your goals, you
may wish to write out your program so you can easily refer to it as you practice.
First, write specific instructions to yourself about the meridian. Second, choose
any of the postures that stimulate the meridian and list them in the order that
you wish to do them. List them in order of difficulty, choosing the easiest one
first. Remember that you do not have to do all of the six postures. One or two
will suffice and you may add the others as you progress. Make your last choice
a seated posture that will enable you to do deep breathing while you work
with the pressure points on your arms, hands, legs or feet. If you have several
health problems or desire to improve your general health, you can eventually
expand your program to include more than one meridian.

Working with Acupressure Points

The diagrams show the whole flow of the meridians. Only five key points have
been identified because these are the only ones you will need to use within the
context of this program. The points identified are the beginning and ending
points of each meridian and the points that specifically stimulate, sedate and
balance the energy within that meridian.

If you have a specific problem to overcome, you should design your program
in a way that allows you to repeat the same exercises each day until your
problem is corrected. Your program should also include postures specifically
designed to balance and relax your body.

Some generalizations that you should consider before you begin working
with Acupressure points include:

1. *How to locate points in general:*   Acupressure points are usually found
    at places where bones intersect, at joints, and in indentations along
    bones or in muscle tissue. When locating a point look for an inden-
    tation on the edge or end of a bone or cartilage. Acupressure points
    are generally somewhat tender with moderate pressure. This is a further
    indication of correct location.
2. *How hard to press:*   Use moderate pressure on areas that are not
    sensitive. On sensitive areas, press only as hard as you can and still
    not cause pain.

3. *How long to press:*   Press for about two minutes. You are working
    with these points as you relax and you may even have your eyes
    closed. There is no need to watch a clock, just relax and estimate
    the time.

4. *Which side to press:*   All pressure points need to be held equally on
    both sides of the body, one side at a time, for an equal length of time.

Visualize the energy flowing through your body on one side at a time or on both sides at once if you can. One side may seem more sensitive than the other. This side of your body is more tense than the less sensitive side. If this happens, hold the pressure on the sensitive side a little longer. The sensitivity will probably lessen or leave altogether as you press.

5. *Which point to choose:* If you have no symptoms, choose the balancing point for continued good health. If you have symptoms refer to the list of common problems in each chapter to decide whether or not you need to stimulate or sedate the point.

Working with Yoga Asanas

Practice Regularly: Even on days when you are too rushed to spend half an hour, choose a few of the asanas and finish with five minutes of deep relaxation.

Never Hurry: Take plenty of time with each of the postures you have chosen to do. The slow, relaxed pace of Yoga will become a lifelong habit and one that will help you in times of stress. Do each asana slowly with maximum concentration.

Body Awareness: Never force the postures. Your exercise should be performed slowly and rhythmically. Avoid forcing a stretch to the point of strain. Your body will know how long to hold the asanas. You may find that your muscles are stiff at first, but after several weeks of practice you will find that your reward will include more supple muscles with better tone. When doing the asanas always try to do them with full awareness and concentration. Read all of the instructions thoroughly before you do the exercise. Do not overdo. Increase the time and degree of each stretch as you go. If you do not feel comfortable with an exercise, such as the Headstand or the Half Lotus Posture, leave it out of your program until you receive instruction from an expert Yoga teacher.

Relaxation: The gentle stretching exercises combined with deep breaths will make you feel relaxed and comfortable as you continue your practice. Deep breathing is an important part of your program and should be included as an integral part of each asana that you do.

Rest in Between the Exercises: Each time you finish an asana, lie on the floor on your back and take deep, relaxing breaths for a minute or two. While relaxing you will become aware of your body's response to each exercise.

Finish with a Five Minute Relaxation: When you have completed your program, add a five minute relaxation that is deep and restful. As you lie on the floor, close your eyes and relax all of the muscles in your body. A short relaxation tape may be helpful; or listening to soft music. Take longer than five minutes if you have the time. Remember, your health and well-being will continue to grow as you practice.

Acupressure combined with Yoga is a total health care system and is beneficial in relieving symptoms of body imbalance. As you continue in your practice your improved health will become more and more evident. With regular practice you can expect the following benefits:

Improved Circulation: You will notice that you have more color in your cheeks and that your hands and feet stay warmer even in cold weather.

Greater Flexibility: As you spine becomes more supple your posture and pose will greatly improve.

Improved Muscle Tone: The rhythmic movements of Yoga will strengthen and tone all of the muscles in your body.

Balanced Organ and Glandular Function: When your major organs and glandular systems function optimally you experience a sense of strength and well-being.

Improved Lung Capacity: The breathing exercises will allow a greater amount of oxygen to be brought to every cell in your body which, in turn, will improve your energy level.

Sounder and More Restful Sleep: The gentle stretching and relaxing exercises of Yoga coupled with the benefits of Acupressure will enable you to fall asleep easily and to awaken feeling fully rested.

Reduced Stress: Acupressure and Yoga are both excellent stress reduction techniques. Practiced together they provide an excellent method for coping with the stressful conditions of daily life.

Detoxification: As your body's ability to eliminate poisons and wastes improves you will discover an increase in your vitality and energy.

Pain Control: Through diligent practice you will find that most painful conditions can be reduced or eliminated.

Rejuvenation: As your bodily functions become more balanced you will notice a lessening of tension wrinkles and lines.

Relaxation: Consistent practice of the relaxation techniques will enable you to relax deeply whenever and wherever you wish.

Prevention of Illness: By learning to use Acupressure and Yoga you can greatly strengthen your body's natural defense systems thereby reducing your chances of illness.

Diagram of the Internal Organs

This diagram will aid you in becoming better acquainted with the location of the Internal Organs of your body.

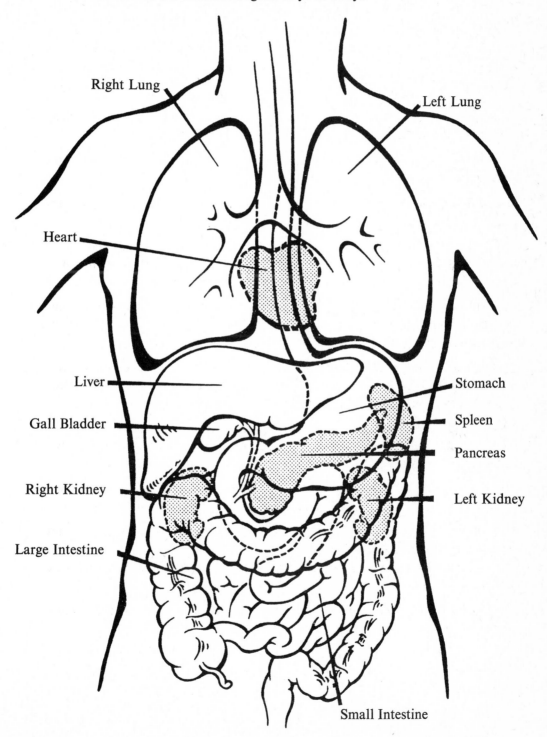

Right Lung

Left Lung

Heart

Liver

Stomach

Gall Bladder

Spleen

Pancreas

Right Kidney

Left Kidney

Large Intestine

Small Intestine

3. *The Warm-up*

It is important to prepare your body with a complete warm-up before you start to work with the asanas. You should start your practice each day with the following sequence of exercises to achieve maximum benefits and to prevent injury.

The Sun Salutation

The slow, stretching movements of *The Sun Salutation* are beneficial for all of the major organs and the endocrine system. The routine invigorates the entire body. The Sun Salutation is traditionally practiced in India in honor of the rising sun, nature's symbol of health and long life. It is a combination of asanas (Yoga postures) that, when mastered, produces a meditative flow of body movement and "wakes up" every cell of the body. The Sun Salutation is a completely balanced series of twelve movements that limber the spine and all of the muscles. The twelve positions in this exercise should be done slowly and rhythmically in a continuous series of stretches. You should concentrate on your breathing and maintain a sense of ease and relaxation as you stretch. You will notice immediate improvement in your flexibility, coordination and circulation. You should start your practice each day with the Sun Salutation. The sequence should be practiced three or more times.

Position 1:   Stand erect with your feet and legs together. Join your palms in the prayer position in front of your chest, with your elbows pointing downward. Exhale slowly.

Position 2:   Keeping your hands close together, slowly raise your arms over your head as you inhale and arch backward. Keep your knees locked and your feet firmly positioned on the floor.

Position 3:   Exhaling, bend forward from the hips, placing your palms down on the floor, on either side of your feet, with your toes and fingertips in a straight line. If this is too difficult, you may bend your knees slightly.

Position 4:   Inhaling, stretch your right leg behind you as far as possible. Rest your right knee on the floor, curl your toes under your foot. Your left foot should remain stationary between your hands. Look forward and arch your back.

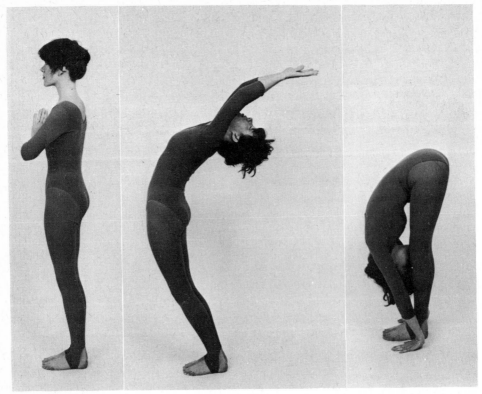

Position 1 **Position 2** **Position 3**

Position 5: Hold your breath as you straighten your right knee and bring your left leg back to join it. Both feet and legs should be together. Straighten your arms with your palms still on the floor so that your entire body forms a straight line (the push-up position).

Position 6: Exhaling, gradually lower your body, touching your knees, chest and forehead to the floor. If it is difficult to place your forehead on the floor you can touch the floor with your chin instead. Your buttocks should remain raised.

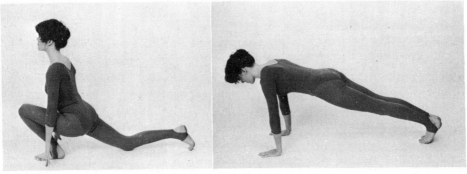

Position 4 **Position 5**

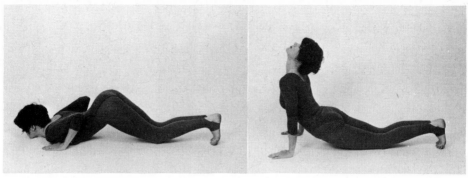

Position 6   **Position 7**

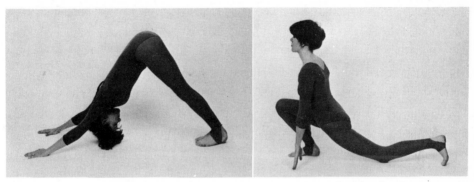

Position 8   **Position 9**

Position 7:   Inhale as you lower your hips and abdomen to the floor, uncurling your toes and relaxing your head, neck and chest. Arch your back and straighten your arms to rest your weight on your hands. The thighs should remain on the floor. Look up and as far back as you can.

Position 8:   Curl your toes under your feet once again. Exhaling, lift your hips, resting your weight on your hands and feet. Your body should form a triangle with your head lowered toward the floor. Keep your feet flat on the floor by pressing your heels down. If this is difficult, walk toward your hands until your feet are flat.

Position 9:   Inhaling, take a long and quick step forward, and place your right foot between your hands. Keep your left leg stretched behind you and lower your left knee to the floor. Then raise your head and arch your back. (This position reverses Position 4.)

Position 10:   Exhaling, bring your left leg forward and place it next to your right leg. Straighten and lock your knees. Place your palms flat on the floor on either side of your feet. Bring your head toward your knees.

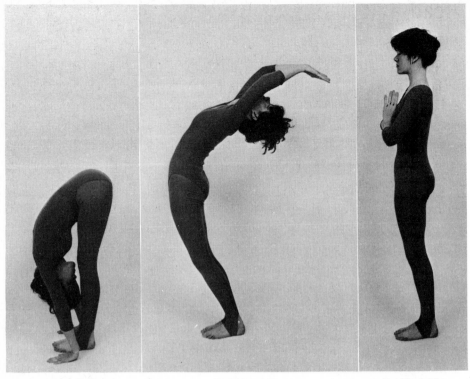

Position 10   Position 11   Position 12

Position 11: Inhale as you slowly stand up, stretching your arms and arching back as in Position 2.

Position 12: Exhaling, gradually lower your arms back to the prayer position. Stand still with your eyes closed for a few seconds. When you are ready, start the sequence again using your left leg as the dominant leg.

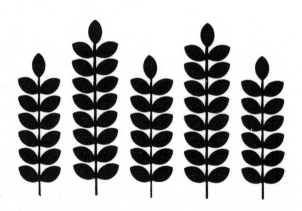

Head and Shoulder Rotation

Sit straight in a cross-legged position or in the Half Lotus Posture. Center your head and spine. Take deep breaths and slowly rotate your head in a large circle to the right. Let it roll freely around. After several rotations change direction and rotate in a large circle to the left. After several rotations, move your head forward and backward. Each motion should be done slowly and accompanied by deep breaths. As your head rolls or moves forward and back use your fingers to massage tension from your neck muscles. When your neck muscles become relaxed, concentrate on your shoulders. Rotate your shoulders in large circles while using your fingers to massage tension and tightness from your muscles.

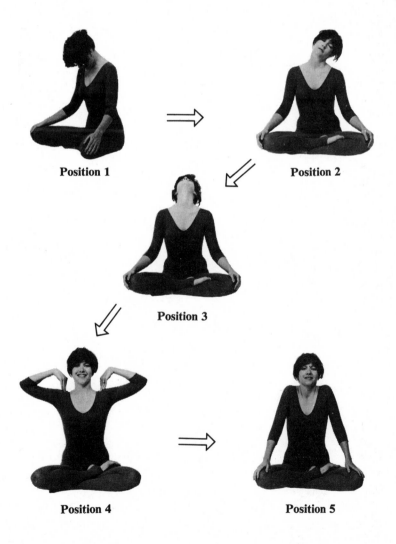

Position 1 **Position 2**

Position 3

Position 4 **Position 5**

Leg and Foot Exercises

Sit on the floor with your legs stretched directly in front of you. Place your hands on your thighs or on the floor slightly behind you. Make sure your posture feels balanced and comfortable. Take deep breaths throughout the exercises.

Exercise 1:   Be aware of your right foot. Flex it, point it and rotate it in large circles. When you are ready, switch to your left foot and do the same exercise. After working with your left foot do the same exercise with both feet at the same time.

Exercise 2:   In the same position, raise your right leg slightly from the floor. Bend your knee and let your foot and lower leg hang down without touching the floor. Rotate your lower leg in large clockwise circles. Change to counter-clockwise circles. Repeat the same exercise with your left leg.

Exercise 3:   Place your right foot on top of your left knee. Slowly stretch your right knee toward the floor and raise it in a "butterfly" motion. Repeat ten times to either side.

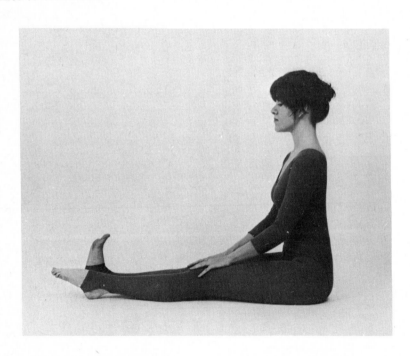

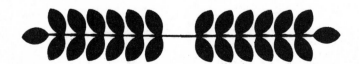

4. The Lung Meridian

The Western Concept: The lungs constitute a key organ for our existence. They are not only the source of oxygen for the combustion of energy inside the body but they also act as an outlet for body poisons and wastes. The lungs exchange oxygen and carbon dioxide through the pulmonary capillaries at the fine membranes where blood and air meet. Lung breathing is the body's external respiration. Internal respiration occurs when each cell takes in oxygen and expels carbon dioxide. Just as proper food is needed for energy and health, deep breathing and good air are vital to life.

The Eastern Concept: In the Eastern tradition, the lungs are called the "tender organ" because they are most easily affected by external influences. It is said that if there is a deficiency of lung energy, the body's resistance to colds and other respiratory diseases will be impaired. Because the lungs administer respiration, they regulate the energy of the entire body. When the lungs are healthy and fully functioning the energy enters and leaves smoothly and respiration is even and regular. A quick and alert mental state also results.

When an imbalance or obstruction impairs either inhalation or exhalation, symptoms such as coughing, asthma, depression or low energy will manifest. The lung meridian energy also controls the health of the skin and body hair. When the lungs are in excellent condition the hair is healthy and shiny and the skin is supple and free from problems.

Pathway of the Lung Meridian: The Lung Meridian begins in the large muscle below the clavicle (collarbone) on the front of the chest. This point has been called "Liberation of Energy" because of its importance in achieving adequate lung ventilation. The meridian energy flows from this point (Lu 1) down the inside or front of the arm and ends at the base of the thumbnail (Lu ll).

Function	Point	Location
Stimulate	Lu 9	To locate this point place the palm of your hand facing you. Look at the crease at your wrist. The point is on the thumb side of that crease.
Sedate	Lu 5	Extend your arm fully with palm facing upward. Bend your arm slightly at the elbow. This point can be found in the indentation on the outside edge of the crease of your elbow.
Balance	Lu 9	Same as the stimulating point.

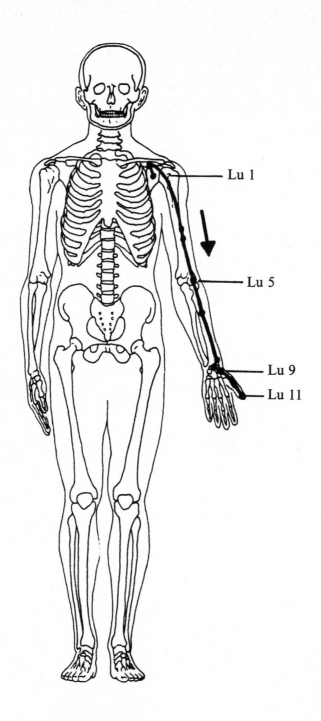

Lung Meridian

Points to Use for Common Problems

Stimulating point Lu 9	Sedating point Lu 5	Balancing point Lu 9
• Sore throat • Chest cold • Low energy • Cold hands • General good health of the lungs	• Tennis elbow • Stiff neck • Shoulder pain • Upper back pain	• Asthma • Dry cough • Chest congestion • General good health of the lungs

To decide whether you need to use the point to stimulate, sedate or balance, look at the chart given above. If you have any of the symptoms listed, choose the point that relates to your imbalance. If you have no specific problem, the balancing point should be used to promote better health. All pressure points should be held equally on both sides of the body for about two minutes on each side.

The following Acupressure points can be pressed while in a cross-legged or Half Lotus Postures. (Page 34)		
To Stimulate:	*To Sedate:*	*To Balance:*
Press: Lu 9 *Then:* Do any of the following 6 postures while visualizing energy flowing from Lu 1 to Lu 11.	*Press:* Lu 5 *Then:* Do any of the following 6 postures while visualizing energy flowing from Lu 11 back to Lu 1.	Do any of the following 6 postures: *Then:* Sit and press Lu 9 (same as stimulating point) while visualizing energy flowing from Lu 1 to Lu 11.

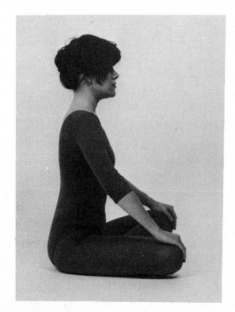

Sit with your spine straight, your mind and body as relaxed as possible and carefully follow the above instructions.

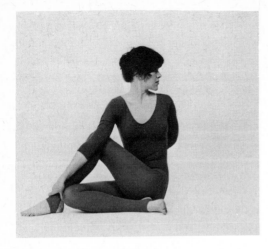

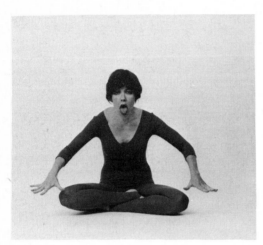

The Spinal Twist: Sit as straight as you can with your legs straight in front of you. Place the right foot flat on the floor outstide the left knee. Place the left arm outside the right leg, and with the left hand hold the right foot or ankle. Beginners may wish to just hold the outside of the right elbow to the outside of the left knee. The right knee should always be as near as possible to the left armpit. Exhale as you turn the body to the right. You may place the right arm behind your back or use it to support you. In either position be sure that your spine is straight. Continue twisting your back and neck as far as you can without strain. Remain in the final pose for a short time while breathing deeply. Slowly return to the starting position. Change legs and repeat to the other side. Practice three times to each side. Try to increase the duration of the stretch. In the advanced pose you may wish to place the left heel against the right buttock.

Lion: Sit in a cross-legged or Half Lotus Position. Inhale through your nose. Remove your hands from your knees and open your eyes as wide as you can. Open your mouth and extend your tongue as far as it will go. Slowly exhale and produce a clear steady "ah" sound from your throat. After your exhalation, return your hands to your knees. Inhale deeply and try to do the next exhalation for an even longer period of time. Do the Lion three to five times.

The Complete Breath: This breathing exercise balances the Lung Meridian. Sit in a Half Lotus Position. Be sure your back is as straight as possible. Begin to slowly exhale through the nose. As you exhale, contract your abdominal muscles and release as much air as you can. Then begin a very slow, quiet inhalation through the nose. At the same time, slowly push out the abdominal muscles which will permit air to enter the lower lung area. When you feel that the abdominal area is distended completely, contract the abdomen slightly and attempt to expand the breath into your chest as far as possible. Raise your shoulders permitting the air to enter the top of your lungs. Hold your breath with your shoulders raised for a count of five. Relax your shoulders and chest as you exhale fully. Contract your abdomen as you exhale. You should make the exhalation as slow and smooth as possible, mentally concentrating on the meridian as you do this breathing exercise. Practice the complete breath frequently. Inhale and exhale very slowly so that you have ample time to complete each section. Perform this exercise three times whenever you become tense or tired throughout the day. With just a few days of practice you will begin to find that this exercise revitalizes your body and brings about a sense of peace and freedom.

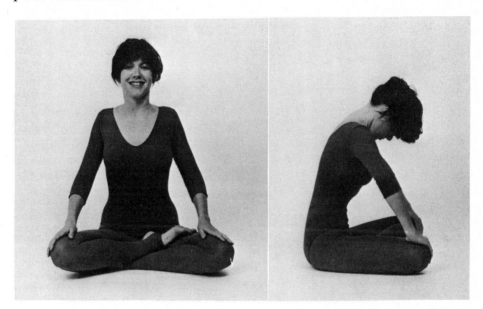

Position 1   Position 2

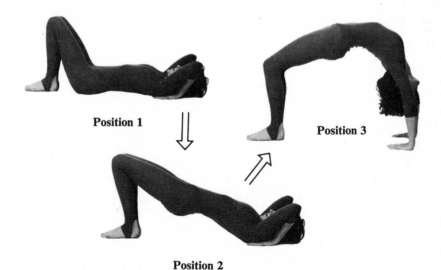

Position 1

Position 2

Position 3

The Wheel: Lie on your back with your knees bent. The feet should be about one foot apart. Arch your back and place the palms of your hands beside the temples with fingers pointing toward the shoulders. Take a deep breath and slowly raise the trunk as you press hard with your arms. Allow the crown of your head to rest on the floor for additional support. The legs will form right angles at the knees. As you continue to straighten the arms and legs your body will raise to form an arch. Breathe slowly while in the Wheel. Exhale slowly as you release the posture. As you release, move slowly back to the head-based and then the supine position. Try to extend the time you hold the posture each time you practice. When you are finished, hug your knees to relax your spine. As you become proficient in this posture you may add slow breaths during the stretch. Repeat up to three times.

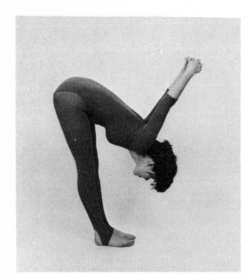

The Double Angle Pose: Stand erect with your feet together. Inhale and extend your arms behind your back and interlock the fingers. Raise your hands as high as you can reach. Bend forward at the waist, exhale while stretching the arms upward. Let your head hang down but attempt to look as far forward as possible. Remain in the final stretch for a short time breathing normally and then slowly return to an erect position. Repeat up to five times.

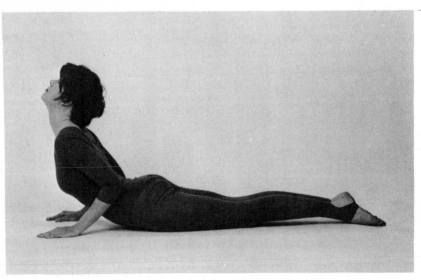

The Cobra: Lie on your stomach with your legs straight. Place your palms flat on the floor under your shoulders. Rest your forehead on the floor and take a deep breath. Exhale as you lift your upper body from the floor. Stretch as far back as you can go without using your arms. Feel the stretch in your back. When you have stretched back as far as possible, add the strength of your arms to lift you further into the stretch. When your arms are straight hold the posture as long as you wish. Breathe normally in the final pose. Be sure to keep your hips close to the floor in this stretch and check to be sure that your legs are still relaxed. Repeat up to five times.

The Bow: Lie flat on your stomach and inhale fully. Bend your knees and grasp your ankles. Be sure that your arms are straight. The strength to hold the bow comes from your arms. Exhale during the preparation and strongly inhale as you arch your back, raise your head, chest and thighs. Stretch as fully as possible. If the initial stretch is easy for you, gently rock back and forth. When you release the posture do so slowly and with caution. Avoid letting go suddenly or snapping out of the asana. The breath may be retained inside in the final pose or slow, deep breathing may be practiced. Repeat up to five times.

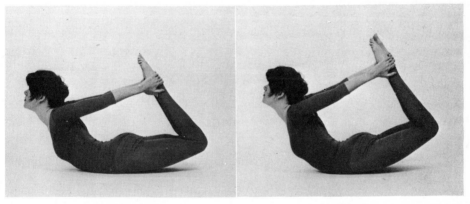

Position 1 **Position 2**

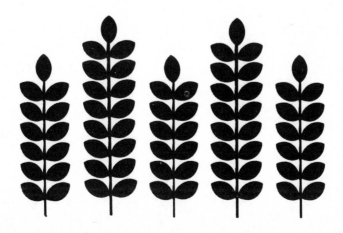

5. The Large Intestine Meridian

The Western Concept: The large intestine's functions are to transform, transport, and to eliminate residues and toxins of digestion and to absorb water and some minerals which have been involved in the digestive process. The waste products of digestion need to be eliminated regularly. A buildup can affect the health of the entire body. The large intestine is a tube about 5 feet in length and is located around the edge of the abdomen in the abdominal cavity. It houses friendly bacteria which help to break down food fiber. At the end of the food's travel through the large intestine a semisolid waste material is left which has a consistency suitable for excretion.

The Eastern Concept: Eastern thought holds that it is especially important to chew food thoroughly. This stimulates the Large Intestine Meridian which goes through the jaws and around the mouth. It is well known that when chewing stops, as in fasting, emptying of the colon also stops. Conversely, vigorous and thorough chewing promotes a complete and healthy function of the large intestine. When waste products accumulate in the colon they produce a toxic effect which affects the mental and physical function of the entire system When waste products are easily eliminated, one experiences a more complete state of health and well-being.

Negative and rigid thought or attitudes also affect the colon by causing it to become constricted and sluggish thereby lowering the energy pattern of the entire body. It is important to regularly include in the diet foods which contain vegetable and whole grain cellulose. These stimulate the large intestine promoting its health, which in turn strengthens the body and spirit.

Function	Point	Location
Stimulate	LI 11	This point is located just at the outside end of the crease of the elbow, against the bone. Find this point by bending your arm and following the crease toward your elbow.
Sedate	LI 2	Clench your fist. This point is located at the base of the index finger, on the side in the indentation on the finger side of the knuckle.
Balance	LI 4	Looking at the back of your hand, locate the point at the base of the web between the thumb and index finger.

The Pathway of the Meridian: The Large Intestine Meridian starts at the inside corner of the index fingernail (LI 1). The energy flows up the back side of the hand and arm to the outside end of the shoulder blade. The flow continues around the shoulder to the front of the body and then ascends the neck, and crosses the midline of the body between the upper lip and the nose ending beside the nostril on the opposite side (LI 20).

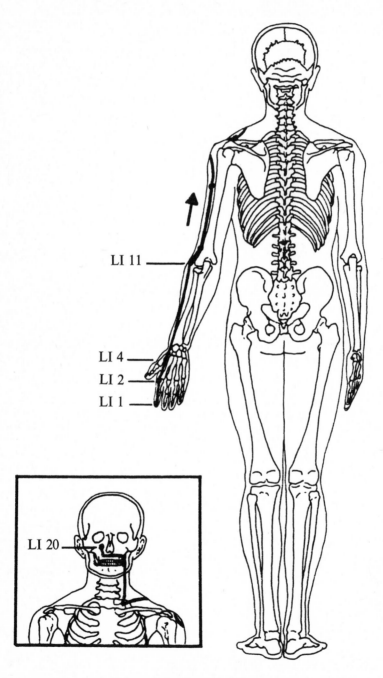

LI 11

LI 4

LI 2

LI 1

LI 20

Large Intestine Meridian

Points to Use for Common Problems

Stimulating Point LI 11	Sedating Point LI 2	Balancing Point LI 4
• Constipation • Nose bleeds • Intestinal gas	• Diarrhea • Prolonged shivering (hard to get warm)	• Regular function of bowels • General good health of large intestine

The following Acupressure points can be pressed while in a cross-legged or Half Lotus Posture. (Page 42)

To Stimulate:	*To Sedate:*	*To Balance:*
Press: LI 11 *Then:* Do any of the following 6 postures while visualizing energy flowing from LI 1 to LI 20.	*Press:* LI 2 *Then:* Do any of the following 6 postures while visualizing energy flowing from LI 20 back to LI 1.	Do any of the following 6 postures. *Then:* Sit and press LI 4 while visualizing energy flowing from LI 1 to LI 20.

To decide whether you need to use the point to stimulate, sedate or balance, look at the chart given above. If you have any of the symptoms listed, choose the point that relates to your imbalance. If you have no specific problem, the balancing point should be used to promote better health. All pressure points should be held equally on both sides of the body for about two minutes on each side.

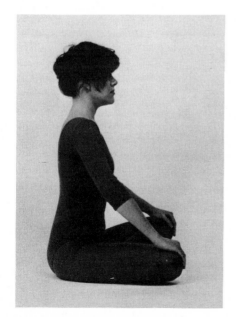

Sit with your spine straight, your mind and body as relaxed as possible and carefully follow the above instructions.

Leg Pulls: Lie flat on your back. Bend your right leg and bring the thigh near the chest. Interlock your fingers and place them over the knee. Inhale deeply and exhale, emptying the lungs. While the lungs are empty, lift the head and upper portion of the chest. Try to touch your knee with your nose. While inhaling, slowly return to the original position. Relax the whole body and then repeat to the other side. For a fuller stretch, straighten and raise one leg at a time. Try to touch your knee with your nose. Repeat five times with each leg.

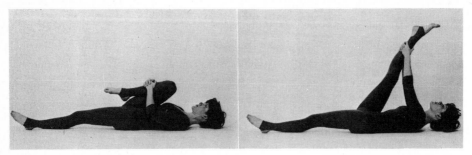

Position 1　　　　　　　　　　　　**Position 2**

The Bow: Lie flat on your stomach and inhale fully. Bend your knees and grasp your ankles firmly with your hands. Be sure that your arms are straight. The strength to hold the bow comes from your arms. Exhale during the preparation and strongly inhale as you arch your back, raise your head, chest and thighs. Stretch as fully as possible. If the initial stretch is easy for you, gently rock back and forth. When you release the posture do so slowly and with caution. Avoid letting go suddenly or snapping out of the asana. The breath may be retained inside in the final pose or slow, deep breathing may be practiced. Repeat up to five times.

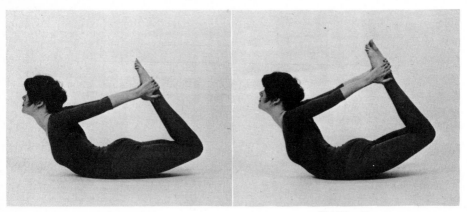

Position 1　　　　　　　　　　　　**Position 2**

The Triangle: Stand with your feet shoulder width apart. Inhale and stretch your arms out to the side. Turn your right foot sideways while keeping your hips centered. Exhale and bring your left arm up and across the midline of your body. Place your right hand on your right knee. Continue the exhalation as you straighten your left arm and bring your right arm down as far as you comfortably can. In the final position, both arms should be in a straight line with your head turned toward your raised hand. Breathe normally while stretching. Hold the stretch for a count of 10 to 15. Inhale while returning to the beginning position. Exhale and be sure your body is centered. Repeat to the other side. Do the stretch five times to each side.

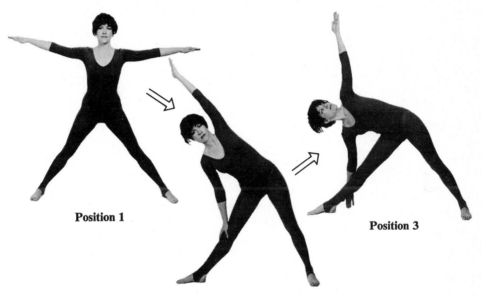

Position 1

Position 2

Position 3

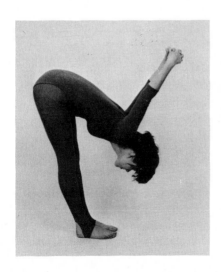

The Double Angle Pose: Stand erect with your feet together. Extend your arms behind your back and interlock the fingers. Raise your hands as high as you can reach. Bend forward at the waist, stretching the arms upward. Let your head hang down but attempt to look as far forward as possible. Remain in the final stretch for a short time and then slowly return to an erect position. Inhale while the arms are forward and when returning to the erect position. Exhale while bending. Repeat up to five times.

The Twisting Cobra: Lie on your stomach with your legs straight. Place your palms flat on the floor under the shoulders. Relax your legs by turning the toes in. Place your forehead on the floor and take a deep breath. Exhale as you lift your upper body from the floor. Stretch as far back as you can go without using your arms. Feel the stretch in your back. When you have stretched back as far as possible add the strength of your arms to lift you further into the stretch. Keep your elbows bent. Slowly twist the upper portion of your body to one side and look at the heel of the opposite foot. Repeat in the other direction. Breathe normally as you stretch. Check to be sure that your legs and hips remain relaxed. Repeat up to five times in each direction.

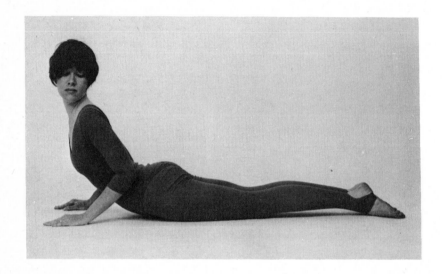

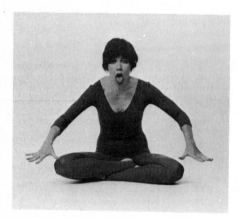

The Lion: Kneel down and lower the buttocks onto your heels. Place your hands on your knees with the palms downward. Tilt your head back, open your mouth and extend your tongue as far as it will go. Open your eyes wide. Inhale through the nose. While slowly exhaling, produce a clear, steady "ah" sound from your throat. Inhale and exhale slowly in unison with the "ah" sound. Do the Lion five times.

6. The Stomach Meridian

The Western Concept: The stomach is in charge of modifying ingested food as part of the digestive process. Since it is centrally located, both physically and functionally (just underneath the left lower ribs), problems of the stomach are quickly reflected in the rest of the body. When food is swallowed it travels to the stomach where it is prepared for further digestion. A valve, called the pylorus, is located at the lower end of the stomach. This valve's function is to open and close rhythmically, allowing food to pass into the small intestine.

The Eastern Concept: In the East, the stomach is described as the "sea of nourishment" or "sea of food and fluid." Differing from the Western idea that the small intestine is the most important organ of digestion, Oriental philosophy considers the stomach to be the primary digestive organ. Food and water are seen to decompose and ripen in the stomach. The elements of food needing no further digestion are sent directly to the spleen which transforms them into the raw material needed for energy and blood. The rest is sent to the small intestine for further digestion and purification.

The natural flow of the Stomach Meridian's energy descends the body. If this energy flow is disturbed or reversed by improper eating or emotional upset, the body reacts with symptoms such as nausea, vomiting, or weakness. The state of one's emotions is closely linked to eating habits and the ability to process food. Being emotionally upset or under stress affects the appetite and nourishment whereas feeling happy and calm stimulates hunger, digestive ability, utilization and appreciation of foods.

The Pathway of the Meridian: The path of the Stomach Meridian starts just below the eye (St 1) and descends to the jaw. A branch outlines the jaw and ascends to the hairline. A second route descends through the collarbone, down the chest and to the pubic area. The flow then veers outward and descends outside the leg to end at the base of the second toenail (St 45).

Function	Point	Location
Stimulate	St 41	Flex your foot. This point is located in the middle of the crease on the front of the ankle in the indentation between the two tendons.
Sedate	St 45	This point is located at the base of the second toenail in the corner toward the outside of the foot.
Balance	St 42	This point is in the center of the foot directly above the second toe.

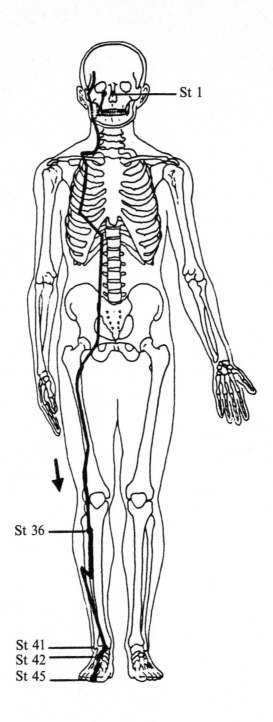

St 1

St 36

St 41
St 42
St 45

Stomach Meridian

Points to Use for Common Problems

Stimulating Point St 41	Sedating Point St 45	Balancing Point St 42
• Low appetite • Nausea • Abdominal bloating	• Always hungry • Always thirsty • Indigestion • Upset stomach	• Stomach gas • Nervousness • Tenseness • General good health of the stomach

The following Acupressure points can be pressed while in a cross-legged or Half Lotus Posture.   (page 48)

To Stimulate:	*To Sedate:*	*To Balance:*
Press: St 41 *Then:* Do any of the following 6 postures while visualizing energy flowing from St 1 to St 45.	*Press:* St 45 *Then:* Do any of the following 6 postures while visualizing energy flowing from St 45 back to St 1.	Do any of the following 6 postures. *Then:* Sit and press St 42 while visualizing energy flowing from St 1 to St 45.

St 45 may be utilized while executing the back stretch.
St 41 and St 42 can be pressed while doing the butterfly.

To decide whether you need to use the point to stimulate, sedate or balance, look at the chart given above. If you have any of the symptoms listed, choose the point that relates to your imbalance. If you have no specific problem, the balancing point should be used to promote better health. All pressure points should be held equally on both sides of the body for about two minutes on each side.

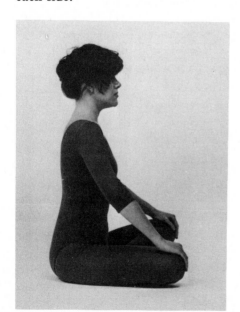

Sit with your spine straight, your mind and body as relaxed as possible and carefully follow the above instructions.

The Cobra: Lie on your stomach with your legs straight. Place your palms flat on the floor under the shoulders. Relax your legs and feet by turning the toes in. Place your forehead on the floor and take a deep breath. Exhale as you lift up from the floor. Stretch as far back as you can go without using your arms. Just feel the stretch in your back. When you have stretched back as far as possible, add the strength of your arms to lift you further into the stretch. When your arms are straight hold the posture as long as you wish. Breathe normally in the final pose. Be sure to keep your hips close to the floor in this stretch and check to be sure that your legs are still relaxed. Repeat up to five times.

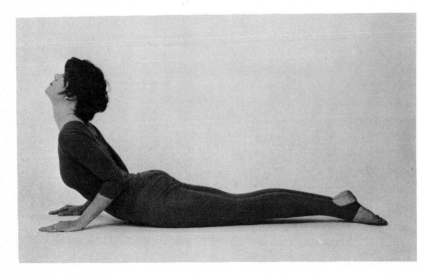

The Bow: Lie flat on your stomach and inhale fully. Bend your knees and firmly grasp your ankles. Be sure that your arms are straight. The strength to hold the bow comes from your arms. Exhale during the preparation and strongly inhale as you arch your back, raise your head, chest and thighs. Stretch as fully as possible. If the initial stretch is easy for you, gently rock back and forth. When you release the posture do so slowly and with caution. Avoid letting go suddenly or snapping out of the asana. The breath may be retained inside in the final pose or slow, deep breathing may be practiced. Repeat up to five times.

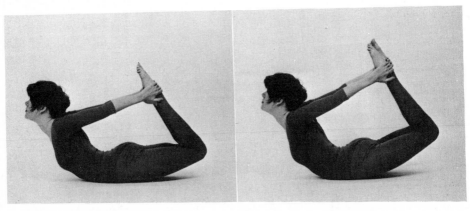

Position 1   **Position 2**

The Back Stretch: Sit on the floor with your legs straight in front of you. Rest your lower arms on your thighs. Relax your entire body, especially the back muscles. Slowly bend forward, sliding your hands along the top of your legs. Try to hold onto your big toes. If this is not possible hold the heels, the ankles or the legs as near to the feet as you can. Continue to relax your back and leg muscles as you stretch. Keep your legs straight and without using the back muscles, only the arms, pull your body a little lower. This should be done gently without any sudden movements or strain. If possible, touch the knees with the forehead. Remain in the final pose for a comfortable length of time, trying to further relax your whole body. Slowly return to the starting position. Be sure your legs are straight throughout the stretch. Exhale slowly while bending forward. Inhale while holding the body motionless. Exhale as you stretch further forward. Breathe fully and deeply in the final stretch. Repeat the stretch five times.

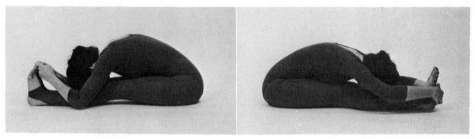

| Position 1 | Position 2 |

The Bridge:

(*Position 1*) Lie on your back with your legs bent at the knees. Raise your back slowly, keeping your feet flat on the floor. Rest your elbows on the floor and support your back with your hands. Inhale as you stretch up and breathe normally during the stretch.

(*Position 2*) When you feel comfortable with Position 1, reach down with your arms to hold your ankles. If you cannot reach your ankles, reach as far as you can. Slowly release the posture by letting go of your ankles and lowering your shoulders, back and buttocks. Hold the posture as long as you comfortably can. You may wish to try Position 1 several times before adding Position 2. Repeat the asana five times.

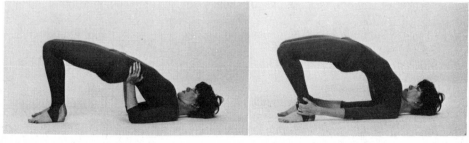

| Position 1 | Position 2 |

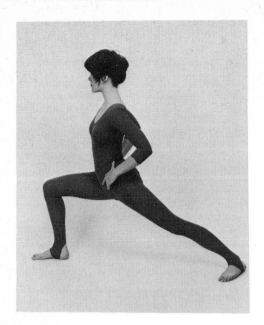

The Hip Stretch: Stand facing forward with your legs placed wide apart. Turn your body sideways. Bend the knee of the front leg while keeping the other leg straight. Make sure that your back is held erect and that your weight is evenly centered between both of your legs. When your right leg is forward, place your hands on your hips. Look forward while maintaining your balance. Hold the stretch for a count of fifteen and then take a deep breath and shift your balance to the other side. Breathe normally during the stretch. Move from side to side slowly and gracefully, alternating the posture. Repeat five times to each side.

The Reverse Boat: Lie on your stomach and stretch your arms out in front of you. Inhale and lift your arms and legs and head as high as you can. Hold your breath during the stretch. Slowly exhale and return to your original position. Repeat five times.

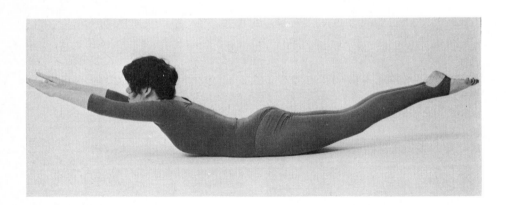

7. The Spleen Meridian

The Western Concept: The Spleen Meridian's energy nourishes the spleen and pancreas but it is traditionally called the Spleen Meridian. The functions of both organs must be considered in order to understand the energy's flow. This meridian also is involved in the health and function of the sexual organs because the spleen meridian's energy passes through them.

The spleen is a purplish-red organ about the size of a fist, located behind the stomach. It is the guardian of the body's complex immunity system. It consists of lymphatic tissue and produces plasma cells which make antibodies. These antibodies in turn, provide protection against various diseases. The spleen acts as a blood reservoir and destroys worn-out red blood cells (about 10 million per second). It also regulates the red blood cells because it is the keeper of iron and hemoglobin.

The pancreas, also located near the stomach, secretes hormones into the blood which regulate the body's use of glucose. Insulin, the pancreas' main hormone, lowers the blood sugar level by stimulating glucose use by the cells. The pancreas also secretes the hormone glucagon which raises the blood sugar level by promoting the conversion of glycogen (by which means carbohydrates are stored in the body) to glucose in the liver. Another function of the pancreas is the secretion of pancreatic enzymes directly into the small intestine which assists in the digestion of fats, proteins and carbohydrates.

The Eastern Concept: The ancient classics say that the Spleen Meridian rules the transformation and transportation of food as well as the balance of liquids in the tissues. The spleen is the crucial link in the process by which food is transformed into energy and blood. If the spleen is unable to activate the processes of food transformation, nourishment and energy are not available throughout the body. The muscles become weak and the lips and mouth become pale and dry. Not only does the spleen help to create blood, it also keeps it flowing in the proper paths. For this reason the Spleen Meridian is the most important meridian associated with menstruation. If the spleen energy is low or unbalanced symptoms such as dismenorrhea, diarrhea, abdominal distension, and excess fatigue may result.

Function	Point	Location
Stimulate	Sp 2	This point is located just below the big toe joint on the side of the foot.
Sedate	Sp 5	This point is just in front of the inner anklebone.
Balance	Sp 3	The location of this point is on the side of the foot just above the large toe joint.

The Pathway of the Meridian: The meridian begins at the base of the large toenail (Sp 1). It travels up the inside of the foot and leg to the groin area. Above the pubic area it ascends the front of the body to the fourth rib. From there it descends to the side of the rib cage where the surface energy ends (Sp 21).

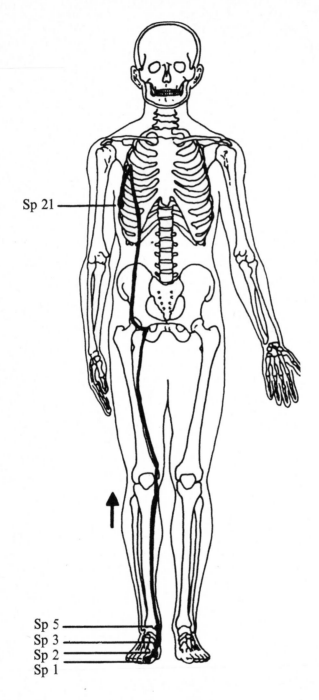

Sp 21

Sp 5
Sp 3
Sp 2
Sp 1

Spleen Meridian

Points to Use for Common Problems

Stimulating Point Sp 2	Sedating Point Sp 5	Balancing Point Sp 3
• Premenstrual bloating • Menstrual aches	• Stomach ache • Tension in knees and thighs • Menstrual pain	• Menstrual irregularity • Sugar imbalance • Constipation • Paleness (iron anemia) • General good health of the spleen and pancreas

The following Acupressure points can be pressed while in a cross-legged or Half Lotus Posture.   (page 54)

To Stimulate:	*To Sedate:*	*To Balance:*
Press: Sp 2 *Then:* Do any of the following 6 postures while visualizing energy flowing from Sp 1 to Sp 21.	*Press:* Sp 5 *Then:* Do any of the following 6 postures while visualizing energy flowing from Sp 21 back to Sp 1.	Do any of the following 6 postures. *Then:* Sit and press Sp 3 while visualizing energy flowing from Sp 1 to Sp 21.

Any of the above points can be utilized while doing the Butterfly Posture or the Alternate Leg Pulls.

To decide whether you need to use the point to stimulate, sedate or balance, look at the chart given above. If you have any of the symptoms listed, choose the point that relates to your imbalance. If you have no specific problem, the balancing point should be used to promote better health. All pressure points should be held equally on both sides of the body for about two minutes on each side.

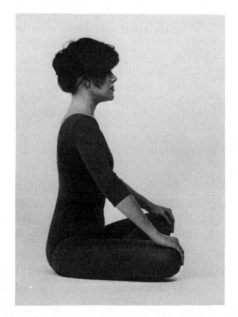

Sit with your spine straight, your mind and body as relaxed as possible and carefully follow the above instructions.

The Butterfly: Sit on the floor and place the soles of your feet together. Sit as straight as you can and try to bring the heels close to your body. Hold onto your feet and gently move your knees toward the floor. When they have reached the maximum stretch, release the pressure and let them come up to your starting position. Establish a slow, steady up and down motion with your knees. Be very careful not to strain the knee joint. Only move your knees as far toward the floor as they comfortably will go. Take deep, relaxing breaths while you practice the asana.

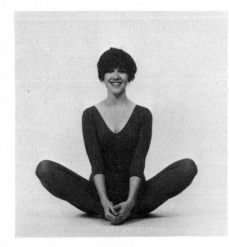 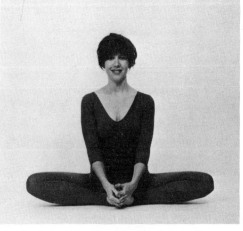

Position 1 Position 2

The Bridge:

(*Position 1*) Lie on your back with your legs bent at the knees. Raise your back slowly, keeping your feet flat on the floor. Rest your elbows on the floor and support your back with your hands. Inhale as you stretch up and breathe normally during the stretch.

(*Position 2*) When you feel comfortable with Position 1, reach down with your arms to hold your ankles. If you cannot reach your ankles, reach as far as you can. Slowly release the posture by letting go of your ankles and lowering your shoulders, back and buttocks. Hold the posture as long as you comfortably can. You may wish to try Position 1 several times before adding Position 2. Repeat the asana five times.

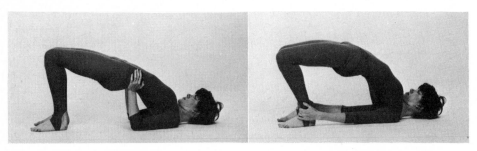

Position 1 Position 2

The Cobra: Lie on your stomach with your legs straight. Place your palms flat on the floor under the shoulders. Relax your legs and feet by turning the toes in. Place your forehead on the floor and take a deep breath. Exhale as you lift up from the floor. Stretch as far back as you can go without using your arms. Just feel the stretch in your back. When you have stretched back as far as possible, add the strength of your arms to lift you further into the stretch. When your arms are straight hold the posture as long as you wish. Breathe normally in the final pose. Be sure to keep your hips close to the floor in this stretch and check to be sure that your legs are still relaxed. Repeat up to five times.

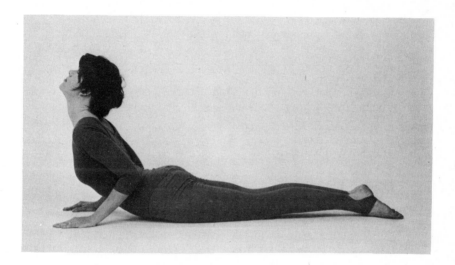

The Locust: Lie on your stomach with your hands under your thighs. Make a fist with each hand. Inhale and raise your legs and stomach as high as possible without bending your knees. Keep your chin on the floor. Hold your breath while you are in the stretch. Exhale while you slowly return to your starting position. Gradually increase the time you are able to hold the stretch (Position 1).

   The Half Locust is done in the same way as the Locust. The legs are alternately raised. If you find the first posture too difficult start with the Half Locust (Position 2). If you can do both postures easily, alternate both five times.

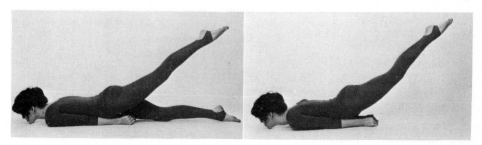

Position 1   **Position 2**

The Boat: Sit on the floor with your legs together and your knees near your chest. Place your hands lightly on the outside on your knees. Take a deep breath and slowly recline back as you extend your legs forward off the floor. Using your arms for balance establish your balance on your buttocks. Try to raise your legs as far as you comfortably can. Keep your arms and legs straight. Maintain the final posture for a short time and then return to the starting position. Rest and repeat three or four times. Try to increase the duration of the stretch as you practice.

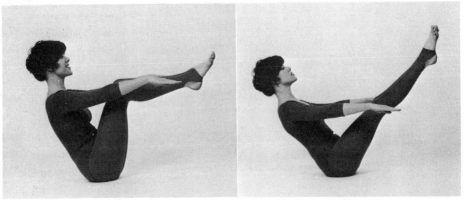

Position 1   **Position 2**

The Alternate Leg Pull: Sit on the floor with your legs stretched in front of you. Fold one leg and place it as far back against the other leg as you can. Exhale and bend forward. Grasp the ankle or toes of the extended leg with both hands. Keep your knee straight. Use your arms to pull your body forward into the stretch until your head is close to your knee. Breathe normally while stretching. Inhale and return to your original position. Repeat three times to each side. Attempt to increase the length of time you are able to remain in the stretch.

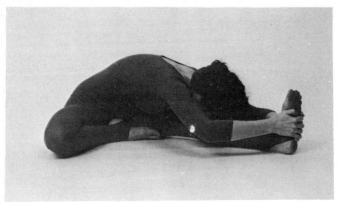

8. The Heart Meridian

The Western Concept of the Meridian: The heart is located just under the breastbone in the center of the chest. It pumps approximately 3,000 gallons of blood per day to the lungs, through which all blood must pass to exchange oxygen and carbon dioxide (a toxic gas that builds up in the bloodstream). The blood is then returned to the heart which pumps it into the arteries to circulate throughout the body.

The action of the heart, with its alternation of tension and relaxation, is a perfect example of the body's need for rest after work. Within a 24 hour day, the heart is at rest for fifteen hours. This supports the yogic principle which provides a period of rest between the stretching or working exercises of *Hatha Yoga.*

The Eastern Concept of the Meridian: In Eastern philosophy the heart is seen to be the "center of the spirit" and the "root of life." It governs and balances the energy of the other organ meridians. The heart, blood and blood vessels are united by their common activity and are mutually interdependent. When the heart and blood energies are balanced, the body and spirit are nourished and the individual lives in harmony with his environment. When these functions are impaired, symptoms such as insomnia, forgetfulness, irrational behavior and depression will result.

The condition of the tongue is closely related to the function of the heart energy. If disharmonies occur in the heart, they are often discernible in the tongue and therefore in the speech. If the heart is functioning normally the face will have a normal complexion and will be moist and bright. If the heart energy is insufficient, the face will become pale and without luster.

The Pathway of the Meridian: The Heart Meridian flow starts deep in the armpit (H 1), ascends the internal front of the arm and curves around to the back of the hand, ending at the inside corner of the small fingernail (H 9).

Function	Point	Location
Stimulate	H 9	Look at the back of your hand. This point is at the base of the little finger-nail on the side closest to the ring finger.
Sedate	H 7	You should never sedate the heart. Use the balancing point.
Balance	H 7	Place the palm of your hand facing you. Look at the crease at your wrist. This point is on the little finger side of that crease.

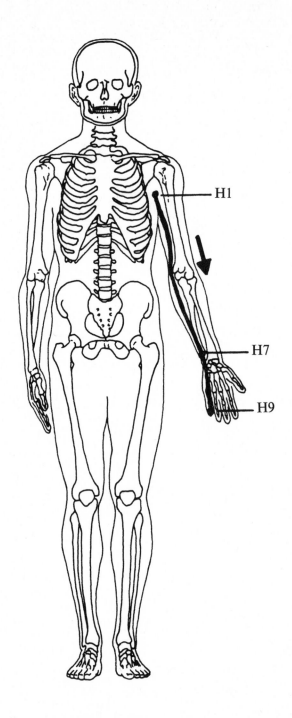

Heart Meridian

Points to Use for Common Problems

Stimulating Point H 9	Sedating Point H 7	Balancing Point H 7
• Low blood pressure • Night sweats • Pale tongue • Yellowish eyes	• There is no sedation point for the heart	• High blood pressure • Insomnia • Excessive thirst • Excessive fear and anxiety • General good health of the heart

The following Acupressure points can be pressed while in a cross-legged or Half Lotus Posture.   (page 60)

To Stimulate:	(*We never sedate the heart energy*.)	To Balance:
Press: H 9 *Then:* Do any of the following 6 postures while visualizing energy flowing from H 1 to H 9.	Use the balancing techniques.	Do any of the following 6 postures. *Then:* Sit and press H 7 while visualizing energy flowing from H 1 to H 9.

To decide whether you need to use the point to stimulate, sedate or balance, look at the chart given above. If you have any of the symptoms listed, choose the point that relates to your imbalance. If you have no specific problem, the balancing point should be used to promote better health. All pressure points should be held equally on both sides of the body for about two minutes on each side.

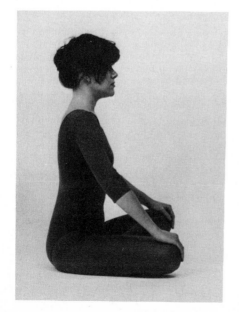

Sit with your spine straight, your mind and body as relaxed as possible and carefully follow the above instructions.

The Pose of A Child: Kneel on the floor. Inhale and start a long, slow exhalation. As you exhale bend slowly forward from the waist and place your forehead on the floor. Bring your hands back by your feet and relax. Remain in the asana, with your eyes closed, for a comfortable length of time while breathing normally. Slowly return to the starting position as you inhale deeply and smoothly.

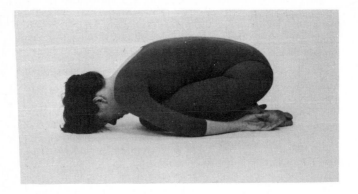

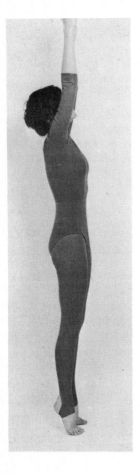

The Heavenly Stretch: Stand as straight as you can with your feet slightly apart. Raise your arms overhead with the fingertips reaching upward and palms facing each other. Look up at your hands. Take a deep breath and hold it while you lift your heels from the floor and stand on tiptoe. Completely stretch the whole body and feel as though you are being drawn upward. Hold the stretch as long as you comfortably can and then slowly exhale as you release the posture. Do the asana five times.

The Cobra: Lie on your stomach with your legs straight. Place your palms flat on the floor under the shoulders. Relax your legs and feet by turning the toes in. Place your forehead on the floor and take a deep breath. Exhale as you lift up from the floor. Stretch as far back as you can go without using your arms. Just feel the stretch in your back. When you have stretched your back as far as possible, add the strength of your arms to lift you further into the stretch. When your arms are straight hold the posture as long as you wish. Breathe normally in the final pose. Be sure to keep your hips close to the floor in this stretch and check to be sure that your legs are still relaxed. Repeat up to five times.

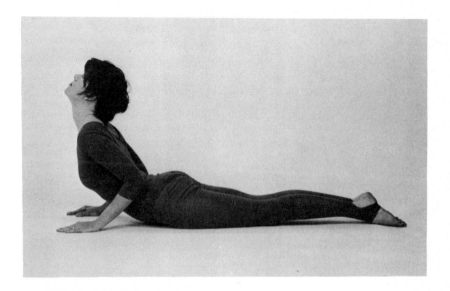

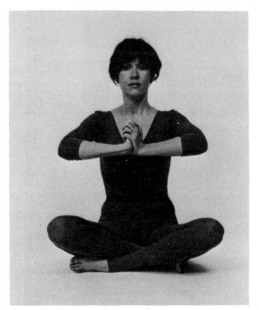

The Arm Strengthener: Sit in the Half Lotus Posture with your head and back erect. Hook your fingers together and hold your hands at chest level. Inhale deeply and pull your arms firmly in opposition. Hold the stretch for a count of five while holding your breath. Exhale and slowly release. Repeat the arm strengthener five times.

The Wheel: Lie on your back with your knees bent. Place your feet about one foot apart. Arch your back and place the palms of your hands beside the temples with fingers pointing toward the shoulders. Take a deep breath and slowly raise the trunk as you press hard with your arms. Allow the crown of your head to rest on the floor for additional support. The legs will form right angles at the knees. As you continue to straighten the arms and legs your body will raise to its fully arched height. Breathe slowly while in the Wheel. Exhale slowly as you release the posture. As you release, move slowly back to the head-based and then the supine position. Try to extend the time you hold the posture each time you practice. When you are finished, hug your knees to relax your spine.

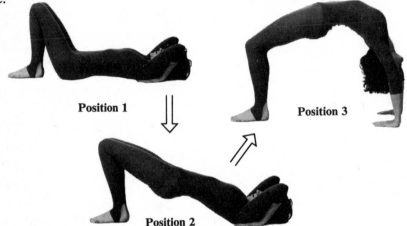

Position 1   Position 3

Position 2

The Plough: Lie flat on your back with your arms beside you. Place the palms of your hands firmly on the floor. Slowly raise your legs over your head. Beginners may need to use their hands and arms for assistance and balance, although you should attempt to keep your legs straight. If this is too difficult, bend your knees and extend your legs back from a bent knee position. Try to touch the floor with the toes of both feet. You may wish to keep your hands on your back for support. If you feel steady in the posture, release your arms or bring them back to touch your toes with your fingers. Breathe slowly and deeply in the asana. Hold your breath when you begin and when you release the posture. Remain in the Plough a comfortable length of time. Try to relax as you stretch. Return slowly to your starting position. Do the Plough two or three times.

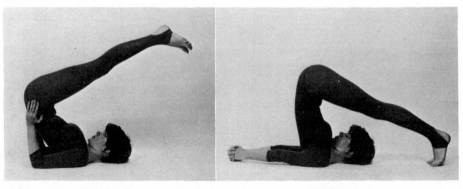

Position 1   Position 2

9. The Small Intestine Meridian

The Western Concept: The small intestine is a coiled tube approximately 23 feet in length which is located in the abdominal cavity. It connects the stomach to the large intestine. Nutrients entering the small intestine are digested and assimilated in this organ. Proper functioning of the small intestine is a major key to complete nourishment. If the small intestine is functioning properly and nutrients move at a reasonable rate, absorption is efficient and waste products are carried on to the large intestine. However, if the small intestine is not functioning properly, the body will receive an inadequate amount of nourishment.

The small intestine chemically changes protein foods into amino acids, complex sugars into simple sugars and fats into fatty acids so that these nutrients are capable of being absorbed. The small intestine also controls the body's store of fluid. It reabsorbs water and passes solid residue on to the large intestine.

The Eastern Concept: The small intestine is the center in which the products of the earth are chemically transformed and absorbed to become a part of the body. The Oriental thought, "man and earth are not two," supports the idea that the condition of the body results from the nutritional value of the earth. From this we can see that the Small Intestine Meridian has a great influence on the body's vitality. The assimilative functions of the Small Intestine Meridian can be seen on the mental level as well as the physical level. Therefore this meridian is also associated with the assimilation of ideas (Food for Thought).

The Pathway of the Meridian: The meridian's route begins at the outside base of the small fingernail (SI 1) and ascends the outer arm to the shoulder. It then zigzags across the shoulder blade before it travels up over the shoulder. From here the energy moves to the base of the neck and up through the cheeks, ending at the front of the ear (SI19).

Function	Point	Location
Stimulate	SI 3	Make a fist. Using your other hand, Press on the end of the largest crease on the outside edge of your hand (underneath your little finger).
Sedate	SI 8	Bend your elbow with your palm facing you. This point is located in the indentation on the inside of your arm just above the point of your elbow.
Balance	SI 4	Look at the back of your hand. This point is located on the little finger side of the back of your hand just before the crease in your wrist.

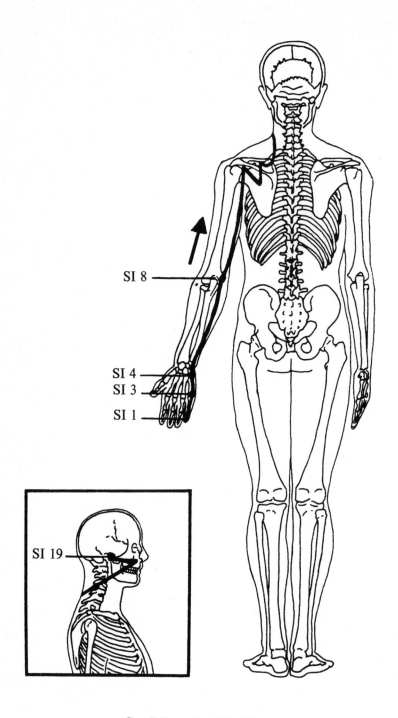

SI 8

SI 4
SI 3

SI 1

SI 19

Small Intestine Meridian

Points to Use for Common Problems

Stimulating Point SI 3	Sedating Point SI 8	Balancing Point SI 4
• Skin irritation • Dry skin • Ringing in the ears • Abdominal distension	• Stiff elbow • Throat spasms • Shoulder pain	• Asthma • General good health of the small intestine

The following Acupressure points can be pressed while in a cross-legged or Half Lotus Posture. (Page 66)

To Stimulate:	*To Sedate:*	*To Balance:*
Press: SI 3 *Then:* Do any of the following 6 postures while visualizing energy flowing from SI 1 to SI 19.	*Press:* SI 8 *Then:* Do any of the following 6 postures while visualizing energy flowing from SI 19 back to SI 1.	Do any of the following 6 postures. *Then:* Sit and press SI 4 while visualizing energy flowing from SI 1 to SI 19.

To decide whether you need to use the point to stimulate, sedate or balance, look at the chart given above. If you have any of the symptoms listed, choose the point that relates to your imbalance. If you have no specific problem, the balancing point should be used to promote better health. All pressure points should be held equally on both sides of the body for about two minutes on each side.

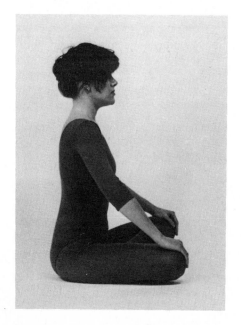

Sit with your spine straight, your mind and body as relaxed as possible and carefully follow the above instructions.

The Triangle: Stand with your feet shoulder width apart. Inhale and stretch your arms out to the side. Turn your right foot sideways while keeping your hips centered. Exhale and bring your left arm up and across the midline of your body. Place your right hand on your right knee. Continue the exhalation as you straighten your left arm and bring your right arm down as far as you comfortably can. In the final position, both arms should be in a straight line with your head turned toward your raised hand. Breathe normally while stretching. Hold the stretch for a count of 10 to 15. Inhale while returning to the beginning position. Exhale and be sure your body is centered. Repeat to the other side. Do the stretch five times to each side.

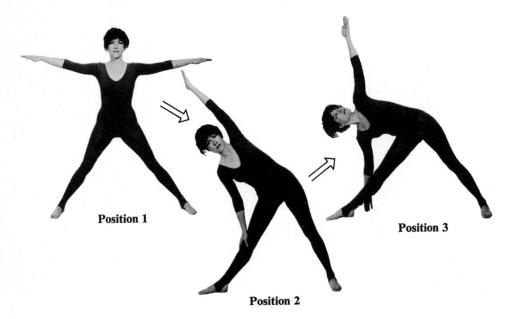

Position 1

Position 3

Position 2

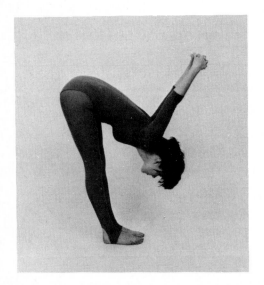

The Double Angle Pose: Stand erect with your feet together. Extend your arms behind your back and interlock the fingers. Raise your hands as high as you can reach. Bend forward at the waist, stretching the arms upward. Let your head hang down but attempt to look as far forward as possible. Remain in the final stretch for a short time and then slowly return to an erect position. Inhale while the arms are forward and when returning to the erect position. Exhale while bending. Repeat up to five times.

The Twisting Cobra: Lie on your stomach with your legs straight. Place your palms flat on the floor under the shoulders. Relax your legs by turning the toes in. Place your forehead on the floor and take a deep breath. Exhale as you lift up from the floor. Stretch as far back as you can go without using your arms. Just feel the stretch in your back. When you have stretched back as far as possible add the strength of your arms to lift you further into the stretch. Keeping your arms bent, twist the upper portion of your body to one side and look at the heel of the opposite foot. Repeat in the other direction. Breathe normally as you stretch. Be sure to keep your hips close to the floor in this stretch and check to be sure that your legs remain relaxed. Repeat up to five times in each direction.

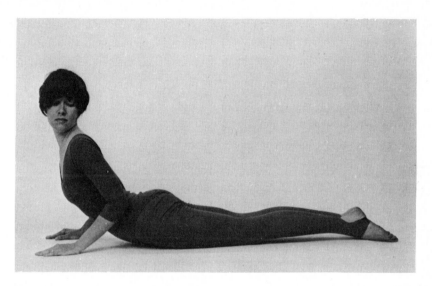

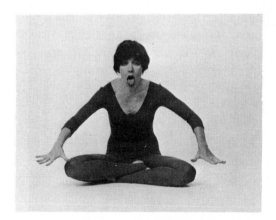

The Lion: Kneel down and lower the buttocks onto your heels. Place your hands on your knees with the palms downward. Tilt your head back, open your mouth and extend your tongue as far as it will go. Open your eyes wide. Inhale through the nose. While slowly exhaling, produce a clear, steady "ah" sound from your throat. Inhale and exhale slowly in unison with the "ah" sound.
Do the Lion five times.

The Wheel: Lie on your back with your knees bent. The feet should be about one foot apart. Arch your back and place the palms of your hands beside the temples with fingers pointing toward the shoulders. Take a deep breath and slowly raise the trunk as you press hard with your arms. Allow the crown of your head to rest on the floor for additional support. The legs will form right angles at the knees. As you continue to straighten the arms and legs your body will raise to its fully arched height. Breathe slowly while in the Wheel. Exhale slowly as you release the posture. As you release, move slowly back to the head-based and then the supine position. Try to extend the time you hold the posture each time you practice. When you are finished, hug your knees to relax your spine. Repeat up to three times.

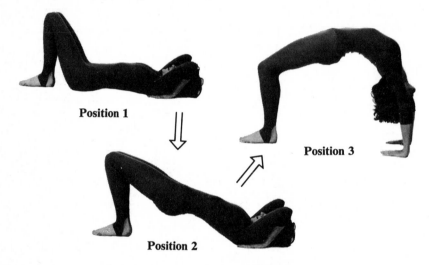

Position 1

Position 2

Position 3

The Bow: Lie flat on your stomach and inhale fully. Bend your knees and firmly grasp your ankles. Be sure that your arms are straight. The strength to hold the bow comes from your arms. Exhale during the preparation and strongly inhale as you arch your back, raise your head, chest and thighs. Stretch as fully as possible. If the initial stretch is easy for you, gently rock back and forth. When you release the posture do so slowly and with caution. Avoid letting go suddenly or snapping out of the asana. The breath may be retained inside in the final pose or slow, deep breathing may be practiced. Repeat up to five times.

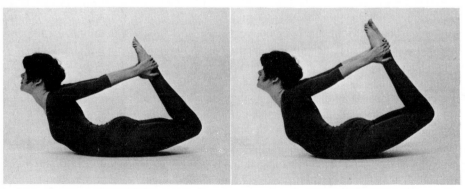

Position 1   Position 2

10. The Bladder Meridian

The Western Concept: The urinary bladder is a hollow muscular sac situated in the pelvis just above the excretory openings. It receives the watery excretion called urine from the kidneys and stores it between urinations. Urine is produced in the kidneys as the end result of cell metabolism from foods and liquids consumed and through respiration. When the bladder is not functioning properly, urinary problems may occur such as incontinence, burning urination, difficulty in urinating or pain in the small of the back.

The Eastern Concept: The energy flow of the Bladder Meridian is extremely complex. This is because of all the many areas of the body that it traverses. The environmental pressures of our society are often responsible for creating an excessive amount of tension which often settles in the back and shoulder areas. This armoring against pressures creates blocks in the flow of the Bladder Meridian energy as the muscles of the back become tense. Because this meridian supplies most of the major organs with energy, it is important to the well-being of the entire body to keep the back muscles supple and the flow of this meridian unblocked.

The Pathway of the Meridian: This meridian is the most complex in its pathway and traverses all parts of the body except the arms. Because of this it also affects most parts of the body. The meridian starts at the inside corner of the eye (B 1), ascends the forehead and goes over the top of the head. It then descends the back in two simultaneous flows. In the buttocks area the flow veers outward and continues down the leg. The two meridian flows intersect at the thigh and join to become a single flow at the back of the knee. Continuing down the back of the leg, the flow then moves behind and below the outside anklebone and finally goes along the outside of the foot to end at the outside base of the little toenail (B 67).

Function	Point	Location
Stimulate	B 67	Locate this point at the outside base of the little toenail.
Sedate	B 65	This point is located halfway between B 64 (see B 64 below) and the base of the little toe on the side of the foot.
Balance	B 64	There is a protruding bone on the outside edge of your foot. This point is located on the little toe side of this protrusion.

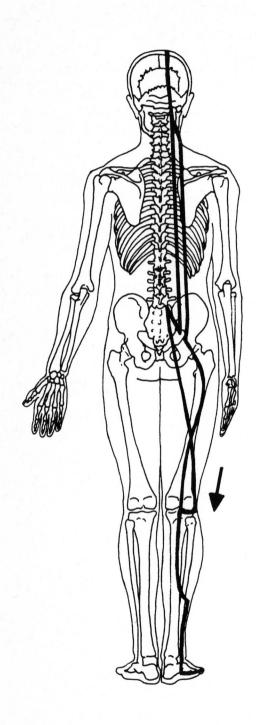
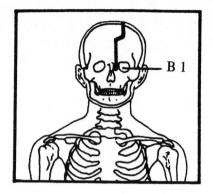
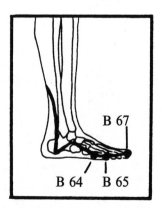

Bladder Meridian

Points to Use for Common Problems

Stimulating Point B 67	Sedating Point B 65	Balancing Point B 64
• Nosebleeds • Runny nose • Frequent urination • Eye problems • Hemorrhoids • Excessive tearing	• Headache • Spinal pain • Spasm or pain in calf muscles • Lower back pain	• To maintain spinal flexibility • General good health of the bladder

The following Acupressure points can be pressed
while in a cross-legged or Half Lotus Posture.   (page 72)

To Stimulate:	*To Sedate:*	*To Balance:*
Press: B 67 *Then:* Do any of the following 6 postures while visualizing energy flowing from B 1 to B 67.	*Press:* B 65 *Then:* Do any of the following 6 postures while visualizing energy flowing from B 67 back to B 1.	Do any the following 6 postures. *Then:* Sit and press B 64 while visualizing energy flowing from B 1 to B 67.

Any of these points can be stimulated while doing
the Alternate Leg Pull.

To decide whether you need to use the point to stimulate, sedate or balance, look
at the chart given above. If you have any of the symptoms listed, choose the
point that relates to your imbalance. If you have no specific problem, the
balancing point should be used to promote better health. All pressure points
should be held equally on both sides of the body for about two minutes on
each side.

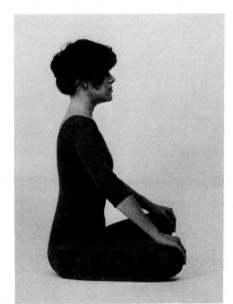

*Sit with your spine straight, your mind
and body as relaxed as possible and
carefully follow the above instructions.*

The Fish: Lie on your back. Using your elbows for support, arch your back and place the crown of your head on the floor. Take a deep breath and accentuate the arch of your back. Breathe deeply and slowly. Remain in the posture for a comfortable length of time. If you feel steady in the posture you may wish to release the elbow support. Put the weight of your upper body onto your elbows to gently release the posture. While in the Fish it is helpful to close your eyes and relax as deeply as possible. Repeat two or three times.

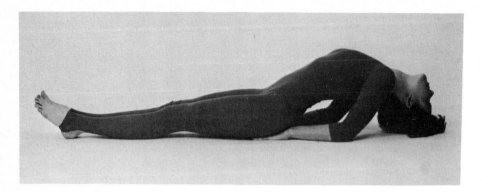

The Cat Stretch: Kneel on the floor with your weight distributed evenly between your arms and legs. Your hands should be flat on the floor and placed directly underneath your shoulders. Inhale, depress your spine and raise your head. Hold for a count of five. Exhale, lower your head and arch your spine. Hold for a count of five. Keep your arms straight and vertical throughout this part of the asana. When you are ready, as you lower your head and arch your back, bring your buttocks slowly back to your heels. Hold for a count of five. Slowly return to your starting position. Do five full rounds.

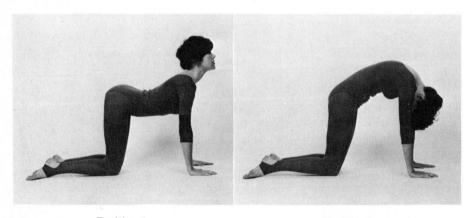

Position 1   **Position 2**

The Alternate Leg Pull: Sit on the floor with your legs stretched in front of you. Fold one leg and place it as far back against the other leg as you can. Exhale and bend forward. Grasp the ankle or toes of the extended leg with both hands. Keep your knee straight. Pull your body forward into the stretch until your head is close to your knee. Breathe normally while stretching. Inhale and return to your original position. Repeat three times to each side. Attempt to increase the length of time you are able to remain in the stretch.

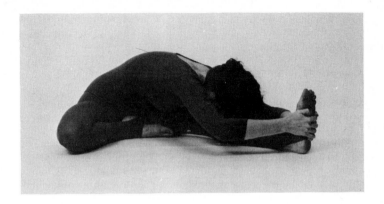

The Spinal Rock: From a seated position, cross your legs and hold onto your toes. Round your back and exhale fully. Gently rock back as far as you comfortably can. Keep your knees bent and your back rounded. Rock back up to your original position, inhaling as you come up. Continue the gentle rocking motion as long as you feel comfortable in the posture. Your legs may extend as far back as is comfortable for you. If you are a beginner, you may wish to start by clasping your hands around your knees. Bring your chin down toward your chest and gently rock back and forth without extending your legs. Rock for a minute or two in either posture.

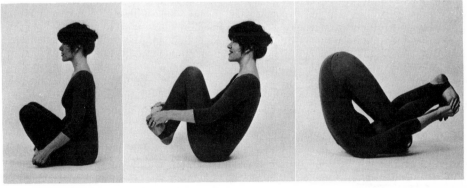

Position 1   Position 2   Position 3

The Plough: Lie flat on your back with your arms beside you. Place the palms of your hands firmly on the floor. Slowly raise your legs over your head. Beginners may need to use the arms for assistance and balance, although you should attempt to keep your legs straight. If this is too difficult, bend your knees and extend your legs back from a bent knee position. Try to touch the floor with the toes of both feet. You may wish to keep your hands on your back for support. If you feel steady in the posture, release your arms or bring them back to touch your toes with your fingers. Breathe slowly and deeply in the asana. Hold your breath when you begin and when you release the posture. Remain in the Plough a comfortable length of time. Try to relax with your eyes closed as you stretch. Return slowly to your starting position. Do the lough two or three times.

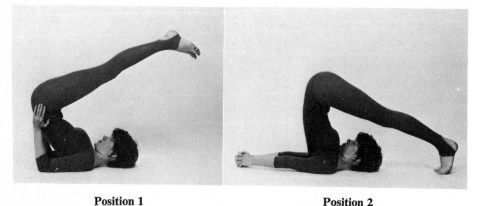

Position 1   Position 2

The Bridge:
(*Position 1*) Lie on your back with your legs bent at the knees. Raise your back slowly, keeping your feet flat on the floor. Rest your elbows on the floor and support your back with your hands. Inhale as you stretch up and breathe normally during the stretch.

(*Position 2*) When you feel comfortable with Position 1, reach down with your arms to hold your ankles. If you cannot reach your ankles, reach as far as you can. Slowly release the posture by letting go of your ankles and lowering your shoulders, back and buttocks. Hold the posture as long as you comfortably can. You may wish to try Position 1 several times before adding Position 2. Repeat the asana five times.

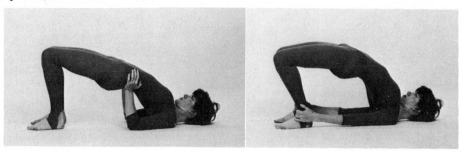

Position 1   Position 2

11. The Kidney Meridian

The Western Concept: The kidney is a very complex organ which regulates the flow of organic waters in the body. It also filters poisons from the blood and acts as a monitor in selecting and reabsorbing the precise amount of proteins, glucose and various minerals needed for correct body functioning. The kidneys are a pair of bean shaped glands situated in the middle of the back on both sides of the spine. They extract many substances from the blood; water, nitrogen compounds such as urea and ammonia, minerals and salts such as sodium chloride, potassium and any other chemicals not needed by the body. Several thousand liters of blood pass through the kidneys daily from which approximately 246 liters of liquid are extracted for further filtering. Most of this liquid is reabsorbed by the body through the kidney's complex filtering system leaving one to two liters to be excreted daily. The kidneys use this large flow of fluid to collect, concentrate, and eliminate the body's wastes.

The Eastern Concept: To the Eastern mind, the kidneys are the "root of life" because they balance and store energy for all of the other organs. This energy is thought to rule birth, development and maturation. As the source of life and individual development, kidney energy is seen to make conception possible, nourish the development of growth to maturity and also is evident in the decline to old age which reflects a weakening of this energy. As time passes, kidney energy decreases in both vitality and quantity, therefore reproductive problems such as sterility or impotence are seen as dysfunctions of the kidney's ability to store and process energy. When the kidneys are deficient in energy, the lower back may become weak and sore, there may be ringing in the ears, and dizziness and night sweats may occur. Other deficient symptoms are loss of energy or warmth, sensitivity to cold, excess fatigue, and muscle weakness especially in the legs.

Function	Point	Location
Stimulate	K 7	Look at the inside of your lower leg. Locate K 3. This point is located two fingers width above K3.
Sedate	K 1	Look at the bottom of your foot. This point is located in line with your middle toe and at the beginning of your instep.
Balance	K 3	Look at your inside anklebone. This point is located halfway between your anklebone and your Achilles tendon.

The Pathway of the Meridian: The Kidney Meridian starts its flow on the sole of the foot (K 1). It crosses the inside edge of the foot and circles behind the inside anklebone. The energy ascends the inside of the leg to the knee. From there it rises to the pubic area. From the genitals it ascends the front of the body to end at the collarbone (K 27).

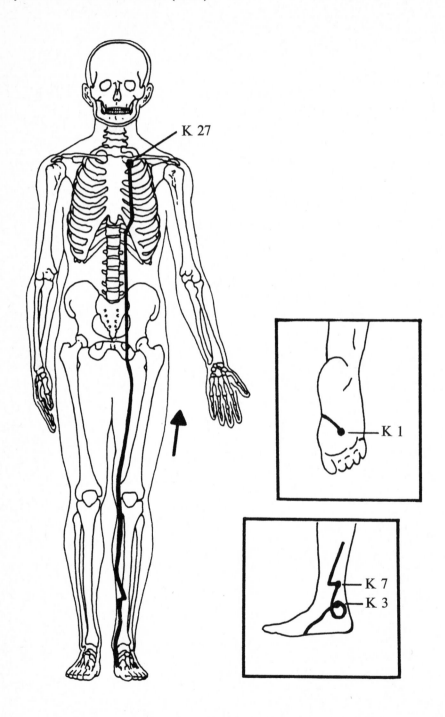

Kidney Meridian

Points to Use for Common Problems

Stimulating Point K 7	Sedating Point K 1	Balancing Point K 3
• Infrequent urination • Weak breathing • Darkness under the eyes • Bloated abdomen	• Soles of feet painful or hot • Too frequent urination • Middle back pain	• Lack of energy • General good health of the kidneys

The following Acupressure points can be pressed
while in a cross-legged or Half Lotus Posture. (Page 78)

To Stimulate:	*To Sedate:*	*To Balance:*
Press: K 7 *Then:* Do any of the following 6 postures while visualizing energy flowing from K 1 to K 27.	*Press:* K1 *Then:* Do any of the following 6 postures while visualizing energy flowing from K 27 back to K 1.	Do any of the following 6 postures. *Then:* Sit and press K3 while visualizing energy flowing from K 1 to K 27.

Any of the above points can be utilized while
doing the Butterfly Posture or the Alternate Leg Pull.

To decide whether you need to use the point to stimulate, sedate or balance, look at the chart given above. If you have any of the symptoms listed, choose the point that relates to your imbalance. If you have no specific problem, the balancing point should be used to promote better health. All pressure points should be held equally on both sides of the body for about two minutes on each side.

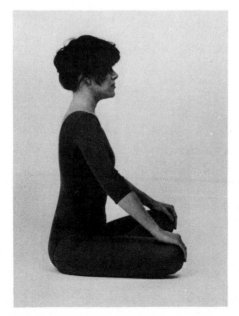

Sit with your spine straight, your mind and body as relaxed as possible and carefully follow the above instructions.

The Butterfly: Sit on the floor and place the soles of your feet together. Sit as straight as you can and try to bring the heels close to your body. Hold onto your feet and gently move your knees toward the floor. When they have reached the maximum stretch release the pressure and let them come up to your starting position. Establish a slow, steady up and down motion with your knees. Be very careful not to strain the knee joint. Only move your knees as far toward the floor as they comfortably will go. Take deep, relaxing breaths while you practice the asana.

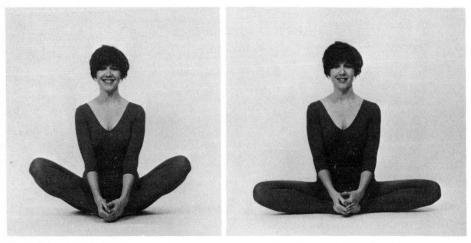

Position 1   **Position 2**

The Alternate Leg Pull: Sit on the floor with your legs stretched in front of you. Fold one leg and place it as far back against the other leg as you can. Exhale and bend forward. Grasp the ankle or toes of the extended leg with both hands. Keep your knee straight. Use your arms to pull your body forward into the stretch until your head is close to your knee. Breathe normally while stretching. Inhale and return to your original position. Repeat three times to each side. Attempt to increase the length of time you are able to remain in the stretch.

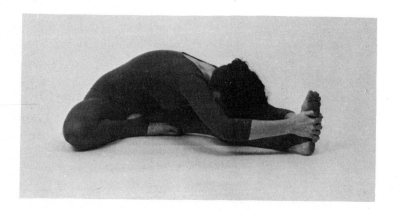

The Bridge:

(*Position 1*) Lie on your back with your legs bent at the knees. Raise your back slowly, keeping your feet flat on the floor. Rest your elbows on the floor and support your back with your hands. Inhale as you stretch up and breathe normally during the stretch.

(*Position 2*) When you feel comfortable with Position 1, reach down with your arms to hold your ankles. If you cannot reach your ankles, reach as far as you can. Slowly release the posture by letting go of your ankles and lowering your shoulders, back and buttocks. Hold the posture as long as you comfortably can. You may wish to try Position 1 several times before adding Position 2. Repeat the asana five times.

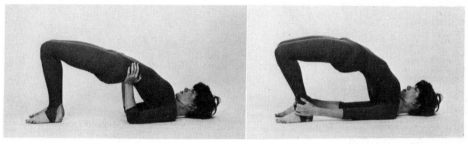

Position 1   **Position 2**

The Cobra: Lie on your stomach with your legs straight. Place your palms flat on the floor under the shoulders. Relax your legs and feet by turning the toes in. Place your forehead on the floor and take a deep breath. Exhale as you lift up from the floor. Stretch as far back as you can go without using your arms. Just feel the stretch in your back. When you have stretched back as far as possible add the strength of your arms to lift you further into the stretch. When your arms are straight hold the posture as long as you wish. Breathe normally in the final pose. Be sure to keep your hips close to the floor in this stretch and check to be sure that your legs are still relaxed. Repeat up to five times.

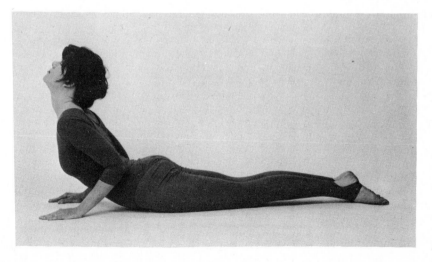

The Locust: Lie on your stomach with your hands under the thighs. Make a fist with each hand. Inhale and raise your legs and stomach as high as possible without bending your knees. Keep your forehead down, close to the floor. Hold your breath while you are in the stretch. Exhale while you slowly return to your starting position. Gradually increase the time you are able to hold the stretch (Position 1).

   The Half Locust is done in the same way as the locust. The legs are alternately raised. If you find the first posture too difficult, start with the Half Locust (Position 2). If you can do both postures easily, alternate both five times.

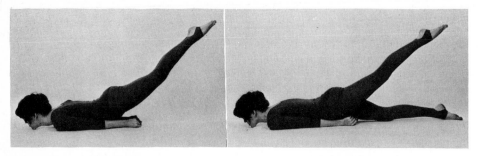

Position 1   **Position 2**

The Reverse Boat: Lie on your stomach and stretch your arms out in front of you. Inhale and lift your arms and legs and head as high as you can. Hold your breath during the stretch. Slowly exhale and return to your original position. Repeat five times.

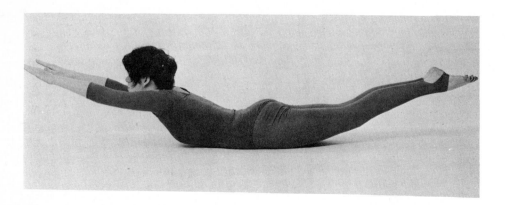

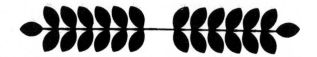

12. The Circulation Meridian

The Western Concept: In Western theory, the Circulation or Pericardium Meridian is so closely related to the heart, that its function and symptomatic problems are treated as part of the overall condition of the heart. The Circulation Meridian and the Heart Meridian both possess the same outward signs to signal trouble, both originate in the same area of the chest. It is important to keep the Circulation Meridian healthy in order to keep the heart healthy. If this Meridian is in a state of imbalance there is a sense of fullness in the chest and sides.

The Eastern Concept: The circulation of life force which connects and unites the organs is ruled by the Circulation Meridian. It is closely connected to the heart and has many of the same danger signals or symptomatic imbalances.

Differing from the other meridians, which are each closely related to a specific organ, the Circulation Meridian is related to several functions. This meridian actually is known by three names which describe the bodily functions it influences. When described as the *Pericardium Meridian*, it is directly correlated with the healthy functioning of the pericardium (the sac holding and protecting the heart). Ancient Eastern thinking states that disease of the heart first affects and weakens the pericardium and thus the energy of its meridian. When described as the Circulation Meridian, its function is to prevent entry of infectious disease into the blood. It is also related to the vascular system and thus influences the circulation. It further regulates the circulation of energy throughout the body, especially in the liver and gall bladder. Lastly, it is called the *Circulation-Sex Meridian* and as such, acts to provide energy for the healthy functioning of the sexual organs.

The Pathway of the Meridian: The meridian flow starts just outside the nipple (C 1). The energy ascends the front of the chest and then turns outward, descending the center of the inside of the arm through the center of the palm and ends at the tip of the middle finger (C 9).

Function	Point	Location
Stimulate	C 9	This point is located at the lower corner of the middle fingernail next to your ring finger.
Sedate	C 7	No sedation point, use balancing point.
Balance	C 7	Look at the palm of your hand. This point is located in the middle of the crease of your wrist.

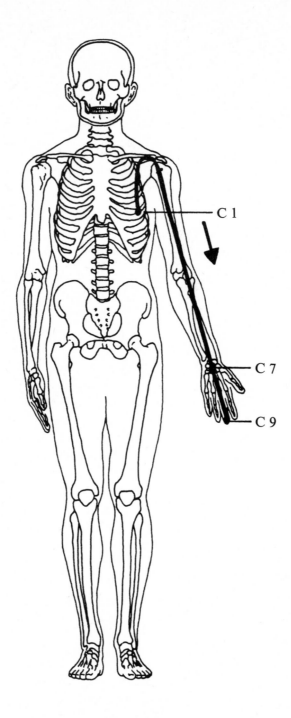

C 1

C 7

C 9

Circulation Meridian

Points to Use for Common Problems

Stimulating Point C 9	Sedating Point C 7	Balancing Point C 7
• Excessive fullness in the chest and sides • Blurred vision	• No sedation point for this meridian	• Laughing excessively for no apparent reason • Menopausal problems • Problems of the reproductive organs • Heart discomfort • Excessively warm hands

The following Acupressure points can be pressed
while in a cross-legged or Half Lotus Posture.   (page 84)

To Stimulate:		*To Balance:*
Press: C 9 *Then:* Do any of the following 6 postures while visualizing energy flowing from C 1 to C 9.	Use balancing techniques in place of sedating circulation energy.	Do any of the following 6 postures. *Then:* Sit and press C7 while visualizing energy flowing from C 1 to C 9.

To decide whether you need to use the point to stimulate, sedate or balance, look at the chart given above. If you have any of the symptoms listed, choose the point that relates to your imbalance. If you have no specific problem, the balancing point should be used to promote better health. All pressure points should be held equally on both sides of the body for about two minutes on each side.

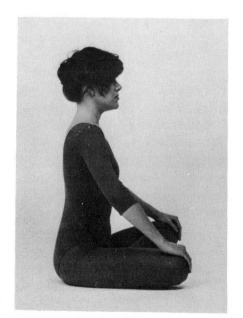

Sit with your spine straight, your mind and body as relaxed as possible and carefully follow the above instructions.

The Cobra: Lie on your stomach with your legs straight. Place your palms flat on the floor under the shoulders. Relax your legs and feet by turning the toes in. Place your forehead on the floor and take a deep breath. Exhale as you lift up from the floor. Stretch as far back as you can go without using your arms. Just feel the stretch in your back. When you have stretched back as far as possible, add the strength of your arms to lift you further into the stretch. When your arms are straight hold the posture as long as you wish. Breathe normally in the final pose. Be sure to keep your hips close to the floor in this stretch and check to be sure that your legs are still relaxed. Repeat up to five times.

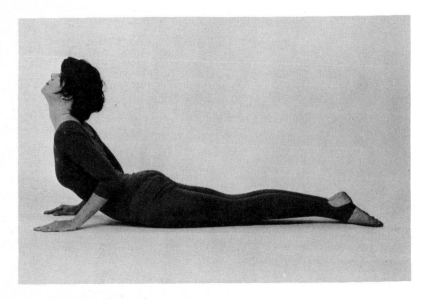

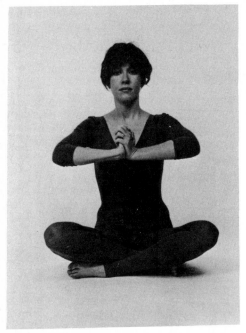

The Arm Strengthener: Sit in the Half Lotus Posture with your head and back erect. Hook your fingers together and hold your hands at chest level. Inhale deeply and pull your arms firmly in opposition. Hold the stretch for a count of five while holding your breath. Exhale and slowly release. Repeat the Arm Strengthener five times.

The Pose of the Moon: Kneel on the floor with your arms at your sides. Inhale and stretch your arms vertically above your head. Exhale and bend forward as you stretch your arms in front of you with your hands and forehead on the floor. Bring your buttocks slowly back toward your heels. Breathe normally for ten seconds, then inhale and bring your arms upward in back of you. Stretch your arms up and back as far as you comfortably can. Interlace your fingers and hold the stretch for a count of five or more if you wish. Breathe normally. Slowly return to your starting position as you exhale slowly. Repeat the asana three times.

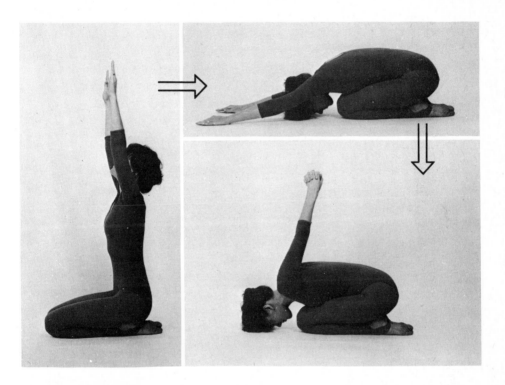

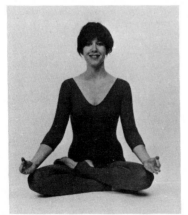

The Half Lotus Posture: Sit on the floor and extend your legs out in front of you. Make sure your back is straight and your head is centered. Hold your left foot firmly and place the sole of your foot next to the inside of your right thigh. The heel of your foot should be placed against the thigh and close to your buttocks. Bring your right foot in and place it on your left thigh or in the fold of your left leg (whichever is more comfortable). Sit erect but not rigid. Rest your hands on your knees unless you are working with the meridian. As you practice take deep breaths. Continue to add to the length of time you are able to remain in the asana. You may wish to reverse the leg position as you practice.

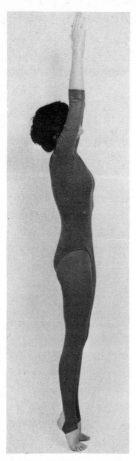

The Heavenly Stretch: Stand as straight as you can with your feet slightly apart. Raise your arms overhead with the palms of your hands facing upward. Look up at your hands. Take a deep breath and hold it while you left your heels from the floor and stand on tiptoe. Completely stretch the whole body and feel as though you are being drawn upward. Hold the stretch as long as you comfortably can and then slowly exhale as you release the posture. Do the asana five times.

The Wheel: Lie on your back with your knees bent. The feet should be about one foot apart. Arch your back and place the palms of your hands beside the temples with fingers pointing toward the shoulders. Take a deep breath and slowly raise the trunk as you press hard with your arms. Allow the crown of your head to rest on the floor for additional support. The legs will form a right angle at the knees. As you continue to straighten the arms and legs your body will raise to its fully arched height. Breathe slowly while in the Wheel.

Exhale slowly as you release the posture. As you release, move slowly back to the head-based and then the supine position. Try to extend the time you hold the posture each time you practice. When you are finished, hug your knees to relax your spine. As you become proficient in this posture you may add slow breaths during the stretch. Repeat up to three times.

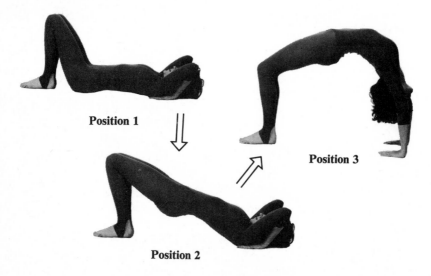

Position 1

Position 2

Position 3

13. The Triple Warmer Meridian

The Western Concept: From the Western point of view the Triple Warmer Meridian is not recognized or used as a part of medical consideration.

The Eastern Concept: The Triple Warmer Meridian relates to a function (as does the Circulation Meridian). It gathers and regulates respiratory, digestive and sexual energy. The organs related to this meridian are the lungs, which are involved with the energy created from oxygen, the small intestine, which changes food and regulates its absorption for caloric energy, and the kidneys, which, along with the Circulation Meridian and Heart Meridian, provide vital life energy. These three divisions of the body are regulated by the meridian's flow. It also works to control body temperature, maintaining warmth in the winter and keeping the body cool during physical exertion and in summer heat. The upper part of the meridian is in control of the lungs, heart and part of the stomach. The middle section unites the stomach, spleen, pancreas, liver and gall bladder. The lower third oversees the small and large intestines, kidneys and bladder.

The Triple Warmer Meridian has been related to a part of the brain called the hypothalamus. This area of the brain (1) regulates body temperature; (2) regulates the autonomic nervous system's emotional response reaction in the internal organs; (3) controls the pituitary gland (the body's master gland) and thereby the entire endocrine system; (4) helps control appetite and thirst; and (5) helps to keep us awake and alert.

The Pathway of the Meridian: The energy of this meridian begins at the base of the fourth fingernail (TW 1) and proceeds up the back of the arm to the shoulder just above the shoulder blade. It then ascends the back of the neck; travels through the mastoid, behind the ear; up around the top of the ear and around to the front of the ear; and finally terminates at the corner of the eyebrow (TW 23).

Function	Point	Location
Stimulate	TW 3	Look at the back of your hand. Find the knuckles at the base of your fourth and fifth fingers. This point is found in the indentation just behind and between these knuckles.
Sedate	TW 10	This point is located just above the point of the elbow toward your shoulder.
Balance	TW 4	Look at the back of your hand. This point is located in the middle of the crease of the wrist.

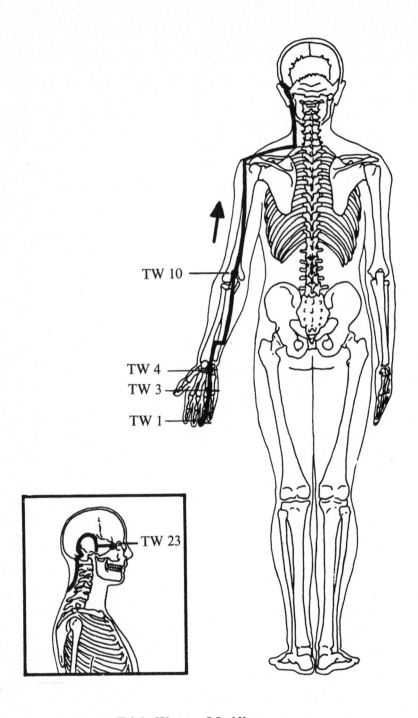

TW 10

TW 4
TW 3
TW 1

TW 23

Triple Warmer Meridian

Points to Use for Common Problems

Stimulating Point TW 3	Sedating Point TW 10	Balancing Point TW 4
• Inability to warm up • Head cold and fever	• Inability to cool down • Cannot straighten elbow • Pain in jaw • Perspiring for no reason • Migraine headaches	• General good health and balance of major body cavity

The following Acupressure points can be pressed while in a cross-legged or Half Lotus Posture. (Page 90)

To Stimulate:	*To Sedate:*	*To Balance:*
Press: TW 3 *Then:* Do any of the following 6 postures while visualizing energy flowing from TW1 to TW 23.	*Press:* TW 10 *Then:* Do any of the following 6 postures while visualizing energy flowing from TW 23 back to TW 1.	Do any of the following 6 postures. *Then:* Sit and press TW 4 while visualizing energy flowing from TW 1 to TW 23.

To decide whether you need to use the point to stimulate, sedate or balance, look at the chart given above. If you have any of the symptoms listed, choose the point that relates to your imbalance. If you have no specific problem, the balancing point should be used to promote better health. All pressure points should be held equally on both sides of the body for about two minutes on each side.

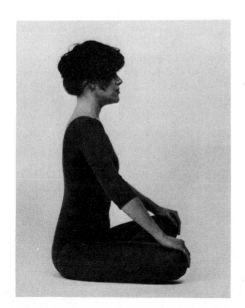

Sit with your spine straight, your mind and body as relaxed as possible and carefully follow the above instructions.

The Triangle: Stand with your feet shoulder width apart. Inhale and stretch your arms out to the side. Turn your right foot sideways while keeping your hips centered. Exhale and bring your left arm up and across the midline of your body. Place your right hand on your right knee. Continue the exhalation as you straighten your left arm and bring your right arm down as far as you comfortably can. In the final position both arms should be in a straight line with your head turned toward your raised hand. Breathe normally while stretching. Hold the stretch for a count of 10 to 15. Inhale while returning to the beginning position. Exhale and be sure your body is centered. Repeat to the other side. Do the stretch five times to each side.

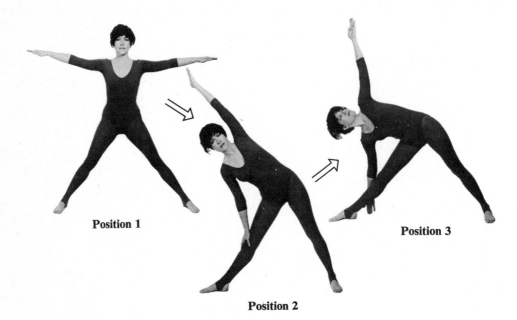

Position 1

Position 3

Position 2

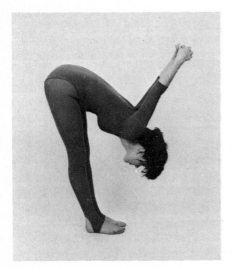

The Double Angle Pose: Stand erect with your feet together. Extend your arms behind your back and interlock the fingers. Raise your hands as high as you can reach. Bend forward at the waist, stretching the arms upward. Let your head hang down but attempt to look as far forward as possible. Remain in the final stretch for a short time and then slowly return to an erect position. Inhale while the arms are forward and when returning to the erect position. Exhale while bending. Repeat up to five times.

The Twisting Cobra: Lie on your stomach with your legs straight. Place your palms flat on the floor under the shoulders. Relax your legs by turning the toes in. Place your forehead on the floor and take a deep breath. Exhale as you lift up from the floor. Stretch as far back as you can go without using your arms. Just feel the stretch in your back. When you have stretched back as far as possible add the strength of your arms to lift you further into the stretch. Keeping your elbows bent, twist the upper portion of your body to one side and look at the heel of the opposite foot. Repeat in the other direction. Breathe normally as you stretch. Be sure to keep your hips close to the floor in this stretch and check to be sure that your legs remain relaxed. Repeat up to five times in each direction.

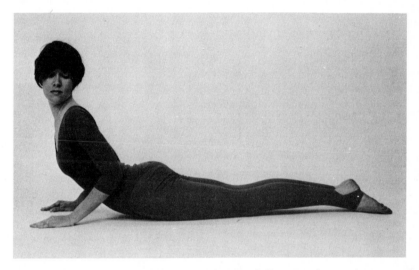

The Bow: Lie flat on your stomach and inhale fully. Bend your knees and firmly grasp your ankles. Be sure that your arms are straight. The strength to hold the bow comes from your arms. Exhale during the preparation and strongly inhale as you arch your back, raise your head, chest and thighs. Stretch as fully as possible. If the initial stretch is easy for you, gently rock back and forth. When you release the posture do so slowly and with caution. Avoid letting go suddenly or snapping out of the asana. The breath may be retained inside in the final pose or slow, deep breathing may be practiced. Repeat up to five times.

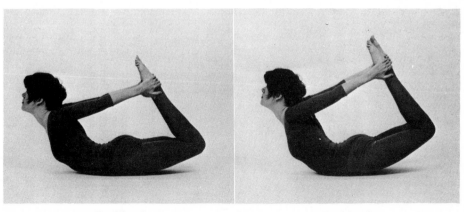

Position 1   **Position 2**

The Wheel: Lie on your back with your knees bent. The feet should be about one foot apart. Arch your back and place the palms of your hands beside the temples with fingers pointing toward the shoulders. Take a deep breath and slowly raise the trunk as you press hard with your arms. Allow the crown of your head to rest on the floor for additional support. The legs will form right angles at the knees. As you continue to straighten the arms and legs your body will raise to its fully arched height. Breathe slowly while in the Wheel. Exhale slowly as you release the posture. As you release, move slowly back to the head-based and then the supine position. Try to extend the time you hold the posture each time you practice. When you are finished, hug your knees to relax your spine.

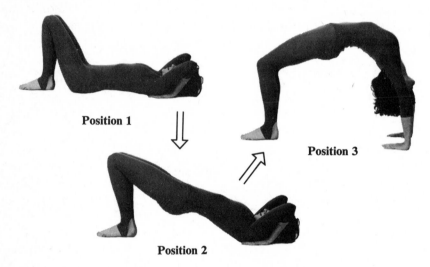

Position 1

Position 2

Position 3

The Bridge:

(*Position 1*) Lie on your back with your legs bent at the knees. Raise your back slowly, keeping your feet flat on the floor. Rest your elbows on the floor and support your back with your hands. Inhale as you stretch up and breathe normally during the stretch.

(*Position 2*) When you feel comfortable with Position 1, reach down with your arms to hold your ankles. If you cannot reach your ankles, reach as far as you can. Slowly release the posture by lowering your shoulders, your back and your buttocks. Hold the posture as long as you comfortably can. You may wish to try Position 1 several times before adding Position 2. Repeat the asana five times.

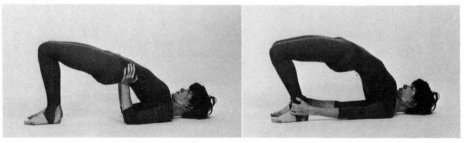

Position 1   **Position 2**

14. The Gall Bladder Meridian

The Western Concept: The gall bladder is a small sac attached to the lower front edge of the central area of the liver. It concentrates, stores and secretes bile used by the body to aid in digestion and elimination. The bile is made up of bilirubin, bile salts, cholesterol, lecithin, fatty acids, electrolytes, and water. During digestion bile is released into the small intestine where it dissolves fats to facilitate their passage through the intestinal wall. It also prevents intestinal putrefaction, contributes to the movement of digesting nutrients and elimination of solid body wastes.

The Eastern Concept: The Gall Bladder Meridian covers all parts of the body except the arms and hands. It zigzags from the back to the front of the body and from the back to the front of the head. Because of this, its energy is involved in many types of imbalances. The condition of the Gall Bladder Meridian can be an indicator of the health of all of the other meridians. It is especially related to various types of headaches, particularly migraines. Blockages can cause pressure and pain in the top of the head, behind the eyes and at the nape of the neck. It is also believed that behavior characterized by anger and rash decisions may be due to an excess of gall bladder energy. Conversely, indecision and timidity may be a sign of gall bladder disharmony or weakness.

The Pathway of the Meridian: The Gall Bladder Meridian begins at the outside corner of the eye (GB 1). It goes down to the corner of the jaw hinge, up to the temple, around the top of the ear and then down to the base of the skull. It then comes back over the head to the forehead and once again drops back down the back of the head. The energy curves around the front of the arm socket, then descends the side of the body, curving forward at the ribs and the hips. It then travels down the outside of the leg, the outside of the foot and ends at the nail of the fourth toe (GB 44).

Function	Point	Location
Stimulate	GB 43	Locate this point one half finger's width above the web between the 4th and 5th toes.
Sedate	GB 38	Locate this point one third of the way up from the outside anklebone toward the side of the knee.
Balance	GB 40	Locate this point on the side of the anklebone toward the center of the foot.

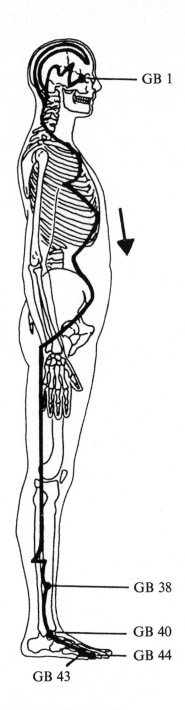

GB 1

GB 38

GB 40

GB 44

GB 43

Gall Bladder Meridian

Points to Use for Common Problems

Stimulating Point GB 43	Sedating Point GB 38	Balancing Point GB 40
• Neck tension • Indecisiveness • Legs weak after sitting • Jaw pain • Headaches (including migraines) • Pain at outer corner of eye	• Irritable • Muscles not limber • Joint pain • Difficulty twisting body	• General good health of the gall bladder

The following Acupressure points can be pressed while in a cross-legged or Half Lotus Posture.   (Page 96)

To Stimulate:	*To Sedate:*	*To Balance:*
Press: GB 43 *Then:* Do any of the following 6 postures while visualizing energy flowing from GB 1 to GB 44.	*Press:* GB 38 *Then:* Do any of the following 6 postures while visualizing energy flowing from GB 44 back to GB 1.	Do any of the following 6 postures *Then:* Sit and press GB 40 while visualizing energy flowing from GB 1 to GB 44.

To decide whether you need to use the point to stimulate, sedate or balance, look at the chart given above. If you have any of the symptoms listed, choose the point that relates to your imbalance. If you have no specific problem, the balancing point should be used to promote better health. All pressure points should be held equally on both sides of the body for about two minutes on each side.

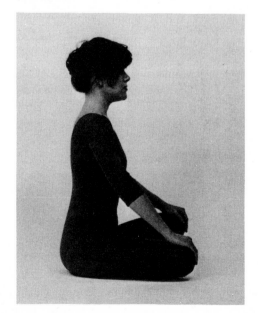

Sit with your spine straight, your mind and body as relaxed as possible and carefully follow the above instructions.

The Spinal Twist: Sit as straight as you can with your legs straight in front of you. Place the right foot flat on the floor outside the left knee. Place the left arm outside the right leg, and with the left hand hold the right foot or ankle. Beginners may wish to just hold the outside of the right elbow to the outside of the left knee. The right knee should always be as near as possible to the left armpit. Exhale as you turn the body to the right. You may place the right arm behind your back or use it to support you. In either position be sure that your spine is straight. Continue twisting your back and neck as far as you can without strain. Remain in the final pose for a short time while breathing deeply. Slowly return to the starting position. Change legs and repeat to the other side. Practice three times to each side. Try to increase the duration of the stretch. In the advanced pose you may wish to place the left heel against the right buttock.

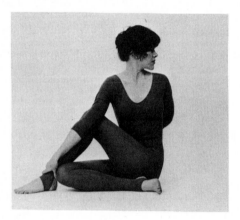

The Bridge:
(*Position 1*) Lie on your back with your legs bent at the knees. Raise your back slowly, keeping your feet flat on the floor. Rest your elbows on the floor and support your back with your hands. Inhale as you stretch up and breathe normally during the stretch.

(*Position 2*) When you feel comfortable with Position 1, reach down with your arms to hold your ankles. If you cannot reach your ankles, reach as far as you can. Slowly release the posture by letting go of your ankles and lowering your shoulders, back and buttocks. Hold the posture as long as you comfortably can. You may wish to try Position 1 several times before adding Position 2. Repeat the asana five times.

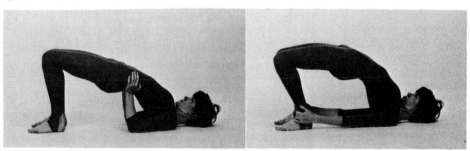

Position 1   Position 2

The Leg Lift: Lie on your right side with the left leg on top of the right leg. Place your right hand under the side of your head and rest on your elbow. Either place your left hand on the floor in front of you for support or, if you do not need support, place it on your thigh. Inhale and raise your left leg as high as you can. When you have your balance, grasp your left ankle and apply a small amount of pressure during the stretch. Keep both of your legs straight. Exhale and lower the leg back to the starting position. Practice the leg lift five times to each side.

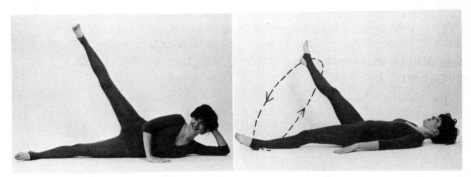

The Leg Lift   **Leg Rotation**

Leg Rotation: Lie flat on your back with your legs straight and the arms beside and in line with your body. Keep your right leg straight as you raise it off the floor and rotate it in a clockwise direction. Rotate it ten times and then change direction and rotate it ten times counterclockwise. Repeat the exercise with the left leg. Be sure that your knees are straight. Your head should remain flat on the floor. Breathe normally during the stretch.

The Cobra: Lie on your stomach with your legs straight. Place your palms flat on the floor under the shoulders. Relax your legs and feet by turning the toes in. Place your forehead on the floor and take a deep breath. Exhale as you lift up from the floor. Stretch as far back as you can go without using your arms. Just feel the stretch in your back. When you have stretched back as far as possible, add the strength of your arms to lift you further into the stretch. When your arms are straight hold the posture as long as you wish. Breathe normally in the final pose. Be sure to keep your hips close to the floor in this stretch and check to be sure that your legs are still relaxed. Repeat up to five times.

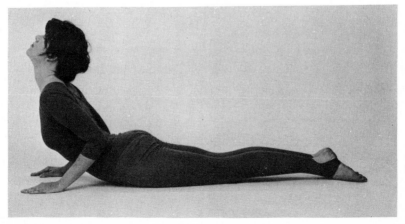

The Headstand: Kneel down and place the forearms on the floor with the fingers interlocked and the elbows in front of the knees. Place the crown of your head between your hands. Hold your hands and head tightly together. Lift the knees off the floor and raise the buttocks until the legs are straight. Slowly walk the legs toward the trunk and allow the knees to bend so that the back is upright with the thighs pressing against the abdomen and lower chest. Slowly transfer the body weight from the toes onto the head and arms. Raise one foot a few inches off the floor. Raise the other foot and balance on the head and arms. When balanced, raise and straighten the hips so that the thighs move up and away from the torso. Straighten your legs. The body should be straight. It may be helpful if you practice against a wall or with someone. Breathe normally. Hold the asana as long as you can. Release the posture gently. Repeat up to three times.

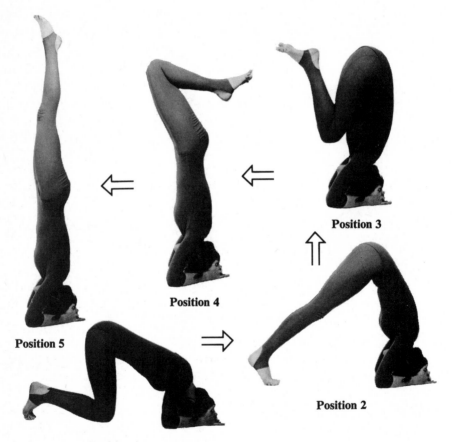

Position 5

Position 4

Position 3

Position 2

Position 1

15. The Liver Meridian

The Western Concept: Located below the diaphragm in the right upper corner of the abdominal cavity, the liver is the largest organ in the body, weighing over three pounds in an adult. Its wedge shape fits the space between the stomach, diaphragm and rib cage. It extends more than halfway across the body. It has a small left lobe and larger right lobe which reaches down to the the level of the lowest rib.

The liver performs approximately 500 bodily functions. It is, therefore, one of the body's most intricate organs. It acts as the body's master laboratory. The liver's most important duties are (1) manufacturing organic compounds such as needed proteins and enzymes; (2) removing dangerous toxic substances from the blood, eliminating poisons such as alcohol, nicotine, caffeine, drugs, sprays and solvents; and (3) storing nutrients to be released into the bloodstream when needed. When muscles need energy, especially after exercise, the liver taps its supply of glycogen, which releases glucose or sugar directly into the bloodstream.

After passing through the spleen, dead red cells are salvaged from the blood by the liver which saves the raw materials to help produce new red blood cells and other body components. Blood clotting substances are also produced by this organ. It manufactures bile which helps to digest fats. Jaundice occurs when the liver malfunctions and bile pigments build up within the bloodstream. This gives the skin and the whites of the eyes a yellow color which is an indicator of liver distress. The liver also helps to balance the hormone, estrogen, which regulates the sex drive and helps control the emotions of depression and anger.

The Eastern Concept: It has been known since ancient times that the healthy flow of energy in this meridian is necessary for spreading and regulating energy throughout the body. The character of the liver is said to be flowing and free. Depression or long-term frustration can upset the function of the organ and result in continuing depression and excessive temper. Because the liver helps control the healthy functioning of the nervous system, a sense of well-being and overall energy is dependent upon the proper functioning of the liver.

All of the organs contribute the purest part of their energy to the eyes, creating the brightness or awareness that characterizes a harmonious spirit. The liver, however, is said to "open into the eyes." Therefore, many disorders of the eyes or the vision are thought to be liver related.

The Pathway of the Meridian: The liver Meridian starts at the inside base of the large toe (Lv 1), travels up the inside of the leg and thigh, and then crosses the pelvis to the outside of the waist. It then flows toward the center and upward, ending between the 6th and 7th ribs (Lv 14).

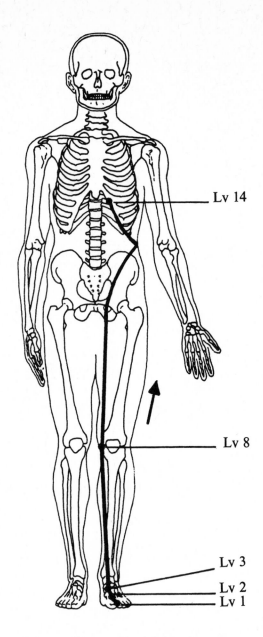

Lv 14

Lv 8

Lv 3
Lv 2
Lv 1

Points to Use for Common Problems

Stimulating Point Lv 8	Sedating Point Lv 2	Balancing Point Lv 3
• Fatigue after mild activity • Soft or cracked nails • Distended chest • Allergies • Distended lower abdomen	• Lower back pain • Muscular spasms or cramps • Belching gas	• Yellowish skin and eyes • General good health of the liver

Function	Point	Location
Stimulate	Lv 8	With the knee flexed, this point can be found on the inside of the leg in the depression at the end of the crease formed by the back of your knee.
Sedate	Lv 2	Look at the top of your foot. This point is located at the web between the big toe and the second toe.
Balance	Lv 3	Look at the top of your foot. This point is located 1 ½ to 2 finger widths above the web between the first and second toes.

The following Acupressure points can be pressed while in a cross-legged or Half Lotus Posture.   (Page 102)

To Stimulate:	*To Sedate:*	*To Balance:*
Press: Lv 8 *Then:* Do any of the following 6 postures while visualizing energy flowing from Lv 1 to Lv 14.	*Press:* Lv 2 *Then:* Do any of the following 6 postures while visualizing energy flowing from Lv 14 back to Lv 1.	Do any of the following 6 postures. *Then:* Sit and press Lv 3 while visualizing energy flowing from Lv 1 to Lv 14.

Any points can be pressed while doing the Butterfly or the Alternate Leg Pulls.

To decide whether you need to use the point to stimulate, sedate or balance, look at the chart given above. If you have any of the symptoms listed, choose the point that relates to your imbalance. If you have no specific problem, the balancing point should be used to promote better health. All pressure points should be held equally on both sides of the body for about two minutes on each side.

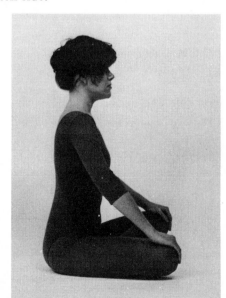

Sit with your spine straight, your mind and body as relaxed as possible and carefully follow the above instructions.

The Butterfly: Sit on the floor and place the soles of your feet together. Sit as straight as you can and try to bring the heels close to your body. Hold onto your feet and gently move your knees toward the floor. When they have reached the maximum stretch, release the pressure and let them come up to your starting position. Establish a slow, steady up and down motion with your knees. Be very careful not to strain the knee joint. Only move your knees as far toward the floor as they comfortably will go. Take deep, relaxing breaths while you practice the asana.

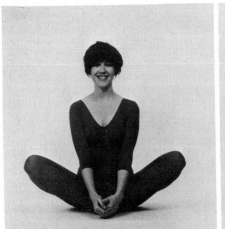 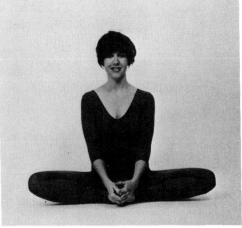

Position 1   Position 2

The Alternate Leg Pull: Sit on the floor with your legs stretched in front of you. Fold one leg and place it as far back against the other leg as you can. Exhale and bend forward. Grasp the ankle or toes of the extended leg with both hands. Keep your knee straight. Use your arms to pull your body forward into the stretch until your head is close to your knee. Breathe normally while stretching. Inhale and return to your original position. Repeat three times to each side. Attempt to increase the length of time you are able to remain in the stretch.

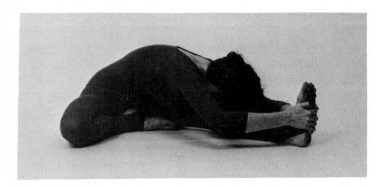

The Locust: Lie on your stomach with your hands under the thighs. Make a fist with each hand. Inhale and raise your legs and stomach as high as possible without bending your knees. Keep your head face down, close to the floor. Hold your breath while you are in the stretch. Exhale while you slowly return to Position 1. Gradually increase the time you are able to hold the stretch.

The Half Locust is done in the same way as the Locust. The legs are alternately raised. If you find the first posture too difficult, start with the Half Locust. If you can do both postures easily, alternate both five times.

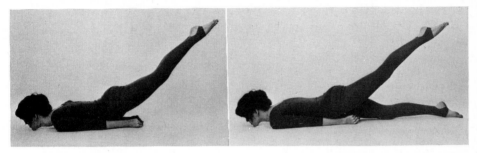

| Position 1 | Position 2 |

The Bridge:

(*Position 1*) Lie on your back with your legs bent at the knees. Raise your back slowly, keeping your feet flat on the floor. Rest your elbows on the floor and support your back with your hands. Inhale as you stretch up and breathe normally during the stretch.

(*Position 2*) When you feel comfortable with Position 1, reach down with your arms to hold your ankles. If you cannot reach your ankles, reach as far as you can. Slowly release the posture by letting go of your ankles and lowering your shoulders, back and buttocks. Hold the posture as long as you comfortably can. You may wish to try Position 1 several times before adding Position 2. Repeat the asana five times.

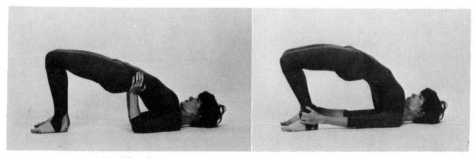

| Position 1 | Position 2 |

The Leg Lift: Lie on your right side with the left leg on top of the right leg. Place your right hand under the side of your head and rest on your elbow. Place your left hand on the floor in front of you for support or place it on your thigh if you do not need support. Inhale and raise your left leg as high as you can. When you have your balance, grasp your left ankle and apply a small amount of pressure during the stretch. Keep both of your legs straight. Exhale and lower the leg back to the starting position. Repeat the leg lift five times to each side.

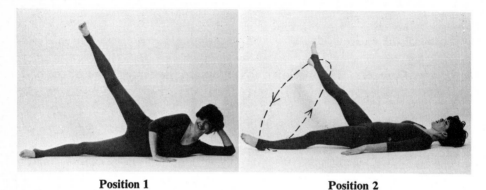

Position 1   **Position 2**

Leg Rotation: Lie flat on your back with your legs straight and the arms beside and in line with your body. Keep your right leg straight as you raise it off the floor and rotate it in a clockwise direction. Rotate it ten times and then change direction and rotate it ten times counterclockwise. Repeat the exercise with the left leg. Be sure that your knees are straight. Your should remain flat on the floor. Breathe normally during the stretch.

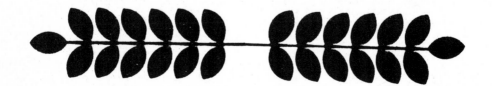

16. The Conception Vessel

(The Great Central Meridian—Front)

The Western Concept: From the Western point of view the Conception Vessel is not recognized or used as a part of medical consideration because its energy flow is not associated with any particular organ but rather functions to balance the energy of the entire body.

The Eastern Concept: The meridian that flows up the center front of the body is called the Conception Vessel. It is frequently described as the regulator of all the meridians on the front of the body. It especially influences the urogenital, digestive and thoracic cavities and the function of the reproductive organs. The meridians of the heart, spleen, lungs, kidneys, liver and circulation receive energy from and give energy to the Conception Vessel. When this meridian is chronically deficient, one tends to be swaybacked.

The Pathway of the Meridian: The energy of the Conception Vessel begins at (CV 1) on the perineum and runs centrally up the front of the body to (CV 24) which is in the depression below the lower lip. (CV 17), on the sternum and between the nipples, is a point that can be used for relaxation. It is pressed by putting the hands together and pressing the backs of the thumbs against the point, as in the Prayer Pose. There are no specific stimulation and sedation points on this energy flow but the energy can be balanced within the flow through meditation. This meridian joins with the Governing Vessel to make a continuous flow of energy in the form of an elongated figure 8 which runs parallel with the spine. The energy pattern of the Conception Vessel, along with that of the Governing Vessel, is extremely important because it aids in balancing and energizing all of the other meridian flows. This in turn helps the energy of the entire body to become evenly distributed.

Note: Working with the Conception Vessel will greatly enhance your practice. These meridians benefit all of the major organs because the meridians associated with the organs travel through either the Front Great Central Meridian or the Back Great Central Meridian. Your practice should always include one or more of the Yoga postures that involve these meridians.

Common problems associated with an imbalance of
the Conception Vessel include:

• Asthma	• Hayfever	• Menstrual problems
• Coughs	• Headaches	• Mouth diseases
• Difficult breathing	• Indigestion	• Pharyngitis
• Eczema	• Influenza	• Pregnancy problems
• Eye problems	• Laryngitis	• Urogenital problems

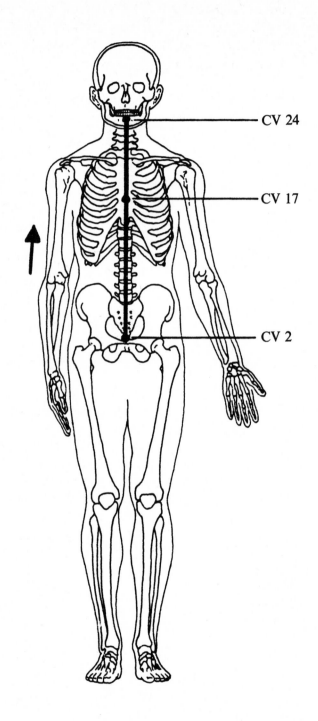

CV 24

CV 17

CV 2

The Conception Vessel: (The Great Central Meridian—Front)

The Locust: Lie on your stomach with your hands under the thighs. Make a fist with each hand. Inhale and raise your legs and stomach as high as possible without bending your knees. Keep your head face down, close to the floor. Hold your breath while you are in the stretch. Exhale while you slowly return to Position 1. Gradually increase the time you are able to hold the stretch.

The Half Locust is done in the same way as the Locust. The legs are alternately raised. If you find the first posture too difficult start with the Half Locust. If you can do both postures easily, alternate both five times.

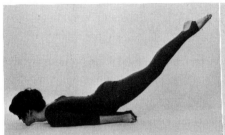 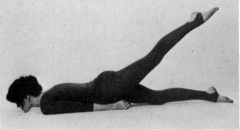

Position 1   **Position 2**

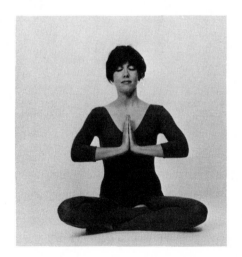

The Prayer Pose: Sit cross-legged or in the Half Lotus Position, Keep your spine erect and your chin and head centered. Hold your hands together and press the knuckles of your thumbs firmly against the meridian point on the sternum which is at the level of your heart. Close your eyes and concentrate on the breath. Send it deeply into this point. Take relaxing deep breaths as you meditate on the energy channel. Feel the calming effect of this centering meditation.

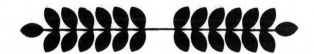

The Wheel: Lie on your back with your knees bent. The feet should be comfortably apart. Arch your back and place the palms of your hands beside the temples with fingers pointing toward the shoulders. Take a deep breath and slowly raise the trunk as you press hard with your arms. Allow the crown of your head to rest on the floor for additional support. The legs will form right angles at the knees. As you continue to straighten the arms and legs your body will raise to its fully arched height. Breathe slowly while in the Wheel. Exhale slowly as you release the posture. As you release, move slowly back to the head-based and then the supine position. Try to extend the time you hold the posture each time you practice. When you are finished, hug your knees to relax your spine. As you become proficient in this posture you may add slow breaths during the stretch. Repeat up to three times.

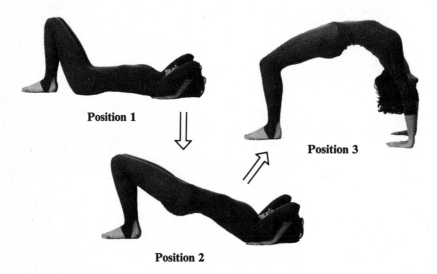

Position 1

Position 3

Position 2

The Reverse Boat: Lie on your stomach and stretch your arms out in front of you. Inhale and lift your arms and legs and head as high as you can. Hold your breath during the stretch. Slowly exhale and return to your original position. Repeat five times.

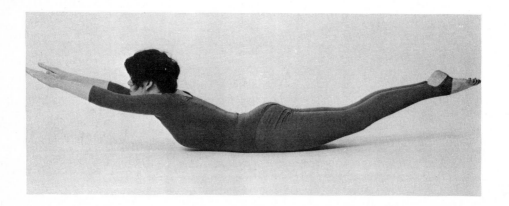

The Cobra: Lie on your stomach with your legs straight. Place your palms flat on the floor under the shoulders. Relax your legs and feet by turning the toes in. Place your forehead on the floor and take a deep breath. Exhale as you lift up from the floor. Stretch as far back as you can go without using your arms. Just feel the stretch in your back. When you have stretched back as far as possible, add the strength of your arms to lift you further into the stretch. When your arms are straight hold the posture as long as you wish. Breathe normally in the final pose. Be sure to keep your stomach close to the floor in this stretch and check to be sure that your legs and hips are still relaxed. Repeat up to five times.

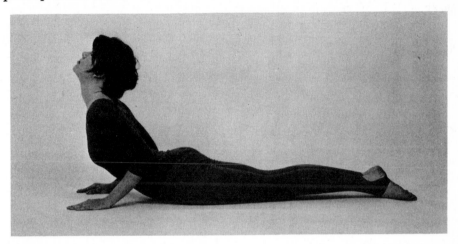

The Bridge:
(*Position 1*) Lie on your back with your legs bent at the knees. Raise your back slowly, keeping your feet flat on the floor. Rest your elbows on the floor and support your back with your hands. Inhale as you stretch up and breathe normally during the stretch.

(*Position 2*) When you feel comfortable with Position 1, reach down with your arms to hold your ankles. If you cannot reach your ankles, reach as far as you can. Slowly release the posture by letting go of your ankles and lowering your shoulders, back and buttocks. Hold the posture as long as you comfortably can. You may wish to try Position 1 several times before adding Position 2. Repeat the asana five times.

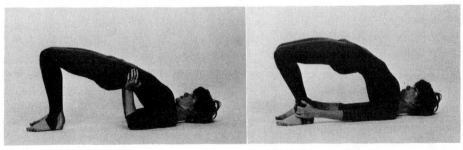

Position 1   **Position 2**

17. The Governing Vessel

(The Great Central Meridian—Back)

The Western Concept: From the Western point of view the Governing Vessel is not recognized or used as a part of medical consideration because its energy flow is not associated with any particular organ but rather functions to balance the energy of the entire body.

The Eastern Concept: The meridian of the Governing Vessel flows up the center of the spine. Its purpose is to provide a sea of energy from which the following meridians and organs may draw: the large intestine, stomach, small intestine, bladder and gall bladder. The energy of the Governing Vessel especially influences the spine and general body energy. When this energy flow is overactive it may result in headaches and pain in the eyes. The spine may also become stiff. When the meridian is chronically deficient in energy, one tends to be round-shouldered and feel heavy-headed. This meridian joins with the Conception Vessel to make a continuous flow of energy in the form of an elongated figure 8 which runs parallel with the spine. The energy pattern of the Governing Vessel, along with that of the Conception Vessel, is extremely important because it aids in balancing and energizing all of the other meridian flows. This in turn helps the energy of the entire body to become evenly distributed.

The Pathway of the Meridian: The meridian of the Governing Vessel begins at the tailbone (GV 1) and ascends the middle of the back along the spine. It goes over the center of the head and down the center of the forehead and nose to end in the center above the upper lip (GV 26). There are no specific stimulation and sedation points on this energy flow.

Note: Working with the Governing Vessel will greatly enhance your practice. These meridians benefit all of the major organs because the meridians associated with the organs travel through either the Front Great Central Meridian or the Back Great Central Meridian. Your practice should always include one or more of the Yoga postures that involve these meridians.

Common problems associated with an imbalance of the Governing Vessel include:		
• Back tension	• Headaches	• Neck pain
• Cold arms and legs	• Hemorrhoids	• Nervousness
• Constipation	• Insomnia	• Urine retention
• Eye problems	• Lower back pain	• Wet cough

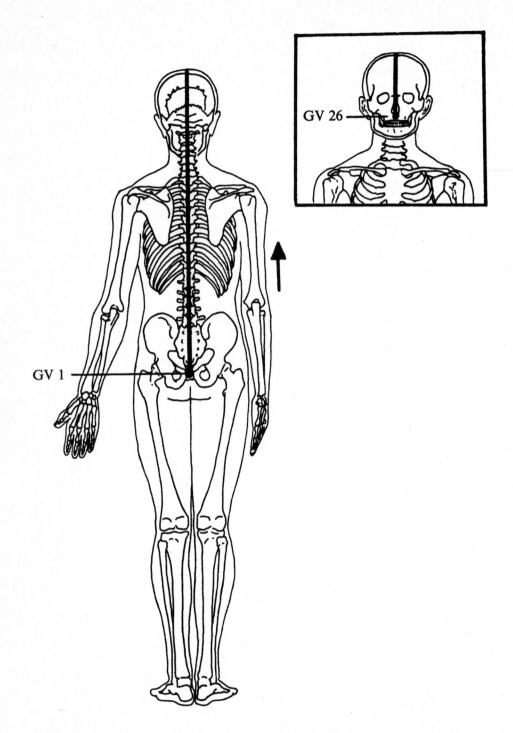

The Governing Vessel: (The Great Central Meridian—Back)

The Cobra: Lie on your stomach with your legs straight. Place your palms flat on the floor under the shoulders. Relax your legs and feet by turning the toes in. Place your forehead on the floor and take a deep breath. Exhale as you lift up from the floor. Stretch as far back as you can go without using your arms. Just feel the stretch in your back. When you have stretched back as far as possible, add the strength of your arms to lift you further into the stretch. When your arms are straight hold the posture as long as you wish. Breathe normally in the final pose. Be sure to keep your hips close to the floor in this stretch and check to be sure that your legs are still relaxed. Repeat up to five times.

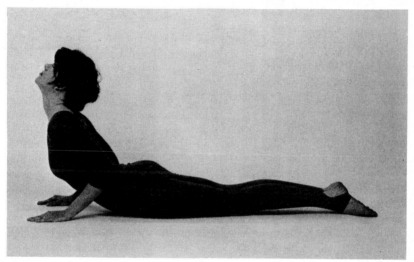

The Bridge:
(*Position 1*) Lie on your back with your legs bent at the knees. Raise your back slowly, keeping your feet flat on the floor. Rest your elbows on the floor and support your back with your hands. Inhale as you stretch up and breathe normally during the stretch.

(*Position 2*) When you feel comfortable with Position 1, reach down with your arms to hold your ankles. If you cannot reach your ankles, reach as far as you can. Slowly release the posture by letting go of your ankles and lowering your shoulders, back and buttocks. Hold the posture as long as you comfortably can. You may wish to try Position 1 several times before adding Position 2. Repeat the asana five times.

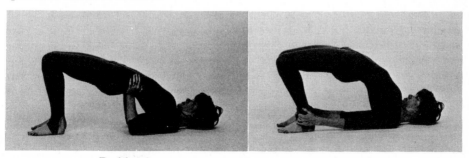

Position 1　　　　　　　　　　　　**Position 2**

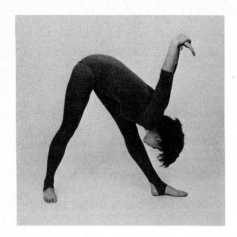

The Head to Toe Pose: Stand straight with your feet about three feet apart. Clasp your hands behind your back and twist your upper body to the left. Bend at the waist while stretching your arms upward. Bring your forehead close to your left leg. Hold the stretch as long as you comfortably can. Slowly release your stretch, return to a standing position and repeat the asana to the other side. You should inhale while standing erect. Retain your breath while twisting, bending and rising. Exhale when returning to a standing position. Repeat five times to each side.

The Spinal Rock: From a seated position, cross your legs and hold onto your toes. Round your back and exhale fully. Gently rock back as far as you comfortably can. Keep your knees bent and your back rounded. Rock back up to your original position, inhale as you come up. Continue the gentle rocking motion as long as you feel comfortable in the posture. Your legs may extend as far back as is comfortable for you. If you are a beginner, you may wish to start by clasping your hands around your knees. Bring your chin down toward your chest and gently rock back and forth without extending your legs. Rock for a minute or two in either position.

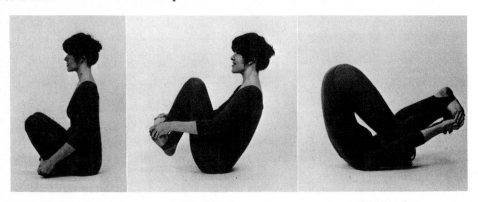

Position 1   Position 2   Position 3

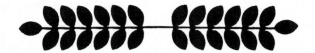

The Shoulder Stand: Lie flat on your back with your feet together. Place your arms at your sides with the palms flat on the floor. Exhale and, using the arms as levers, raise the legs and back to a vertical position. Bend your elbows and use your arms for support. Steady your back with the palms of your hands; fingers should be pointing up in the center of your back. Hold your body as straight as you can. Flex your feet. Try to form a right angle as your legs extend upward; the neck and chest press against the chin. Breathe normally when steadied in the raised position. Exhale and release the posture gently when you are ready. If the full Shoulder Stand is too difficult, do the inverted posture (Position 1). Hold your body at a 45 degree angle to the floor instead of a right angle. Repeat up to three times.

Increase your endurance by holding the posture a few seconds longer each day.

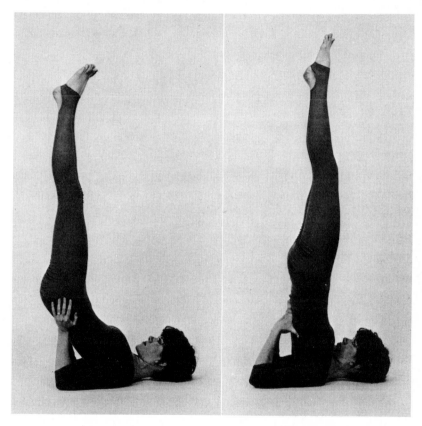

Position 1   **Position 2**

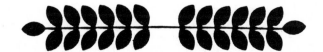

The Headstand: Kneel down and place the forearms on the floor with the fingers interlocked and the elbows in front of the knees. Place the crown of your head between your hands. Hold your hands and head tightly together. Lift the knees off the floor and raise the buttocks until the legs are straight. Slowly walk the legs toward the trunk and allow the knees to bend so that the back is upright with the thighs pressing against the abdomen and lower chest. Slowly transfer the body weight from the toes onto the head and arms. Raise one foot a few inches off the floor. Raise the other foot and balance on the head and arms. When balanced, raise and straighten the hips so that the thighs move up and away from the torso. Straighten your legs. The body should be straight. It may be helpful if you practice against a wall or with someone. Breathe normally. Hold the asana as long as you can. Release the posture gently. Repeat up to three times.

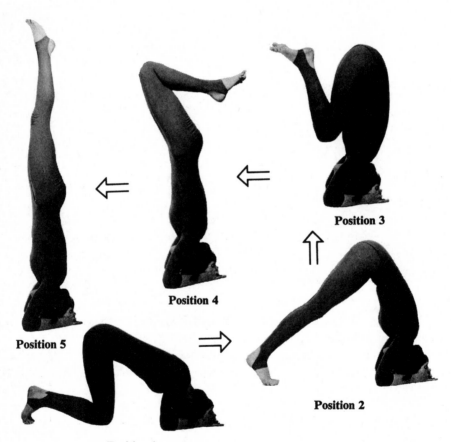

Position 5

Position 4

Position 3

Position 2

Position 1

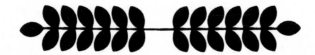

Glossary

Achilles tendon—The strong tendon joining the muscles in the calf of the leg to the bone of the heel.

Acupressure—A system of health care which stimulates the flow of body energy by applying pressure to specific points on the body.

Acupuncture—A system used by the Chinese whereby fine needles are inserted along the meridians to balance the energy flow of the body.

Allergies—An excessive reaction to substances, situations, or physical states that usually do not affect the average individual.

amino acids—The building blocks of protein.

antibodies—The substances that neutralize body toxins.

Arjuna—Central figure and warrior-hero of the *Bhagavad Gita*. Devotee and friend of Lord Krishna.

armoring—The body's muscular reaction to tension which leads to a contracting and squeezing of muscles.

asana—A steady Yoga posture.

assimilation—The taking in of new ideas; the receiving of nourishment by the body.

autonomic nervous system—Part of the nervous system that governs involuntary action of the body.

balance—To bring into harmony.

Bhagavad Gita—One of the essential scriptures of Hinduism, a portion of the *Mahabbarata*, in which Lord Krishna instructs Arjuna on the nature of God, universe and Self.

Bhakti Yoga—Concentration and meditation on the Divine Principle.

bilateral—On both sides of the body.

bile—The fluid manufactured by the liver that is stored and secreted by the gall bladder to aid in the digestion of fats.

blockage—Congestion of energy at an Acupressure point.

Body awareness—An understanding and awareness of one's mental, emotional and physical health.

breastbone—The sternum or central bone in the front of the upper chest.

caloric energy—The energy derived from the digestion and absorption of foodstuffs.

capillaries—Very small blood vessels.

carbon dioxide—The waste material eliminated from the lungs in exhalation.

cartilage—Connective tissue.

chakra—Anatomically identified with the nerve plexuses of the body. Vital for receiving life energy.

chi—The Chinese term for vital energy.

circulation—Movement in a regular course throughout the body.

clavicle—The bone connecting the shoulder with the breastbone; sometimes called the collarbone.

Concentration—The act or process of centering one's complete attention on a single object.

Conception Vessel—The channel of energy which travels up the front of the body from the perineum or the base of the torso to the space between the upper lip and the nose. This channel is a major flow for the energy needed to nourish the body's organs.

Detoxification—The act of removing poisons or the effect of poisons from one's body.

dharana—Concentration.

dhyana—Contemplation.

diaphragm—A body partition of muscle and connective tissue, found in the upper abdominal cavity. Necessary for respiration.

digestion—The breaking down of food for assimilation into the system.

disease—A lack of balance in the body causing symptomatic conditions.

Do-in—A form of Acupressure that is self-administered.

endocrine system—A system of ductless glands which secrete hormones throughout the body.

energy—A dynamic force which is the basis of all living forms. It travels throughout the body in systematic paths called meridians.

estrogen—A hormone secreted by the ovaries.

feces—Solid waste matter to be eliminated from the body.

first aid point—A pressure point useful for temporary measures.

Flexibility—A suppleness or elasticity of the human body whereby muscles and joints are capable of bending with ease.

G-jo—A form of first-aid acupressure to relieve specific symptoms.

gland—An organ in the body that manufactures a substance to be used by the body.

glucose—The simple sugar found in the blood.

glycogen—Sugar stored in the liver.

Governing Vessel—The channel of energy which travels up the back of the body from the tailbone at the base of the spine, over top of the head and ends at the point between the upper lip and the nose. This channel is a major flow for the energy needed to keep the muscles supple and the body in a healthy state.

Hatha yoga—Yogic stretching and strengthening exercises.

hemoglobin—The iron containing pigments of the red blood cells which carries oxygen from the lungs to the tissues.

hormones—Secretions of the endocrine system, which stimulate or alter bodily functions.

hypothalamus—A part of the brain which includes autonomic regulatory centers.

I Ching—Known as *The Book of Change*, it has been used by the Chinese to explore the meaning of human affairs for thousands of years.

instep—The arch middle portion of the foot in front of the ankle joint.

insulin—A secretion of the pancreas which controls the blood sugar level.

intuition—Immediate understanding of a given situation without complete and rational knowledge of that situation.

Japa Yoga—The repetition of a phrase.

jaundice—An accumulation of bile in the blood causing a yellowness of the skin and whites of the eyes.

Jin-shin—A form of Acupressure using both hands to balance energy in all areas of the body.

Jnana Yoga—The Yoga of knowledge.

karma—The universal law of cause and effect.

Karma Yoga—The Yoga of action.

ki—The Japanese term for vital energy.

Krishna—In Hindu philosophy, a form of God incarnated.

kundalini—Life energy residing at the base of the spine which travels upward during spiritual awakening.

Laya Yoga—The Yoga of devotion or absorption.

lymphatic system—A system which carries certain nutrients and removes wastes from the cells throughout the body.

mantra—Words repeated during meditation to still the mind and bring about higher states of consciousness.

Mantra Yoga—A repeated phrase.

mastoid—A protrusion of the skull located behind the external ear.

meditation—Directing one's attention inward. Contemplation of the Universal Self.

membrane—A thin, soft, flexible layer of tissue found in the body.

meridian—A specific flow of energy within the body connecting Acupressure points and internal organs.

meridian flow—The direction of energy flow in the body.

Mukusha—A Yogic ideal of unification.

muscle tone—An indicator of the capability of the body's musculature for healthy and vigorous performance.

organic compounds—Compounds contributing to or affecting living organisms.

organic waters—Body water and fluid.

oxygen—An element found in the air as an odorless, colorless, tasteless gas essential to life.

Patanjali—A learned Indian teacher who wrote the Yoga Sutras in the 2nd Century B.C.

pelvis—Bowl shaped structure that supports the soft internal organs of the lower abdomen; formed by the hip bones on each side.

pericardium—The sac holding the heart to protect it from shock.

perineum—The base of the torso in the area between the anus and the exterior genitalia.

pituitary—The master endocrine gland of the body controlling various internal secretions.

plasma cells—The cells found in the watery part of blood and lymph.

posture—A held stretch used in Yoga.

prana—The Indian term for vital energy.

pranayama—Breathing exercises and breath control leading to deep relaxation and used to enhance the Yoga asanas.

pressure point—A point on the body that is most receptive to the alteration of the body's energy.

program—A planned set of actions.

protein—An important nourishing substance that is found in all plant and animal cells.

pubic bone—A bone in the lower front section of the pelvis.

pulmonary—Relating to, functioning like, or associated with the lungs.

putrefaction—The decomposition of organic matter.

pyloral valve—The valve at the lower end of the stomach which controls the types and quantity of food which enters the small intestines.

Raja Yoga—The Yoga of mind control.

red blood cells—The cells which carry iron and oxygen to the body cells.

rejuvenation—To restore to a healthy or vital state of health. To make youthful.

relaxation—The state of physical calm.

respiration—The act of breathing which oxygenates the living tissues of the body.

Samadhi—The highest state of attainment in Yoga in which the yogi transcends the physical and mental limitations of the body.

Sanskrit—The classical language of ancient India.

sedate—To calm; to withdraw excessive, blocked energy.

self-discipline—The regulation of one's behavior for the sake of improvement.

Shiatsu—A form of Acupressure practiced in Japan.

Shiva—The king of Yogis.

sternum—The breastbone.

stimulate—To arouse, to tonify a deficient area.

stress—Tensions which alter the physiological and mental balance in man.

Swami Vivekananda—Introduced Yoga to the United States in approximately 1900.

thorax—That part of the body between the neck and the abdomen containing the heart and lungs.

tonify—To stimulate; to bring energy to a deficient area.

toxins—Poisons found in the body.

urine—The liquid containing wastes of the body.

urogenital organs—The organs of excretion and reproduction.

vascular system—The channels carrying blood throughout the body.

Vedas—Ancient Hindu scriptures.

vital energy—The energy that provides living things with the substance for life.

warm-up—Movement designed to increase the body's capacity for exercise.

yang—The active principle of energy.

The Yellow Emperor's Classic—The study of Acupuncture/Acupressure written 4,000 years ago in what is thought to be the first medical book ever written.

yin—The passive principle of energy.

Yoga—The science of well-being originating in India.

Yoga Sutras—Written by Patanjali in the 2nd Century B.C., a scholarly writing which describes the complete system of Yoga.

Yogi—In India, a student of Yoga.

Yukta—One in common with God.

Bibliography

Acupressure

Chang, Dr. Stephen Thomas, *The Complete Book of Acupuncture*, Millbrae, Calif., Celestial Arts Publications, 1976

Gach, Michael Reed, *Acu-Yoga*, Tokyo, Japan, Japan Publications, Inc., 1981

de Langre, Jacques, *Do-In 2*, Magalia, Cal, Happiness Press, 1976

Lawson-Wood, Denis and Lawson-Wood, Joyce, *Five Elements of Acupuncture and Chinese Massage*, Rustlington, Sussex, England, Health Science Press, 1975

Teeguarden, Iona, *Acupressure Way of Health: Jin shin do*, Tokyo, Japan, Japan Publications, Inc., 1978

Wollerton, Henry and McLean Colleen, *Acupuncture Energy in Health and Disease*, Wellingborough, Northamptonshire, England, Thorsons Publishers Ltd., 1979

Yoga

Couch, Jean and Weaver, Nell, *Runners World Yoga Book*, Mountain View, Cal., Runners World Books, 1982

Hewitt, James, *The Complete Yoga Book*, New York, Schocken Books, 1978

Hittleman, Richard, *Yoga, a twenty-eight day exercise plan*, New York, Workman Publishing Co., 1974

Iyengar, B.K.S., *The Concise Light on Yoga*, New York, Schocken Books, 1982

Kent, Howard, *A Color Guide to Yoga*, Maidenhead, Berkshire, England, Intercontinental Book Productions, 1980

Index